"Well, let me at least walk you back."

"I'm fine, really."

"If you get bored and want someone to talk to over the next few weeks, I'm here every Tuesday evening with my fellow louts."

"I'll keep that in mind," Claire said, truly appreciative of his offer.

Kiernan's lips curved into a slight grin. "Oh—and one more thing. If you decide to hit up the usual tourist spots, you might want to spray down the Blarney Stone with a strong antiseptic before kissing it. Just saying."

Claire chuckled quietly. "That's good advice."

Kiernan smiled and nodded. "Well, you take care."

"You, too." Claire said as she walked past him.

Once outside, she took a deep breath and allowed the cool night air to seep into her lungs. For a split second, she questioned her decision to close the door on any further interaction with Kiernan. But she had no choice. She had come to Ireland to make a difficult decision that could potentially alter the course of her life from here on out. The last thing she needed was to tempt another complication that would only create more heartache. She had had enough of that for a lifetime already.

Dear Reader,

I've always assumed that doctors are adept at separating their personal and professional lives. But what would happen if one were to experience a personal trauma so closely tied to their field of medicine, they could no longer fully engage in their career? That was the question that led to the premise of *Healing the Baby Surgeon's Heart*.

Unable to fully recover emotionally from the stillbirth of her daughter, Dr. Claire Delaney, an ob-gyn from Boston, has come to Ireland for a month to figure out if she can regain the passion she once felt for her profession. What she doesn't expect to find is a strong attraction to Dr. Kiernan O'Rourke, the handsome, rugby-playing chief of surgery whose dedication to his career leaves no room for relationships or children. Or so he thinks. But love has a way of shifting priorities...and healing hearts.

I hope you enjoy reading Claire and Kiernan's story as much as I enjoyed writing it!

Tessa

HEALING THE BABY SURGEON'S HEART

TESSA SCOTT

MEDICAL ROMANCE

Harlequin®
MEDICAL ROMANCE

Recycling programs
for this product may
not exist in your area.

ISBN-13: 978-1-335-94285-2

Healing the Baby Surgeon's Heart

Harlequin Enterprises ULC
22 Adelaide St. West, 41st Floor
Toronto, Ontario M5H 4E3, Canada
www.Harlequin.com

Printed in U.S.A.

Tessa Scott is a lover of animals, nature and happily-ever-afters. She lives in Northeast Connecticut surrounded by lots of trees, wildlife and a menagerie of pets. A copywriter by day, she enjoys that magical moment when the characters she creates come to life and help take the story in new and exciting directions.

Healing the Baby Surgeon's Heart
is Tessa Scott's debut title for Harlequin.

Visit the Author Profile page at Harlequin.com.

In memory of my mom, who always
encouraged me to follow my dreams.

CHAPTER ONE

CLAIRE DELANEY PULLED her soft cardigan tight around her chest as a breeze rose off the Atlantic Ocean and flitted through her thick chestnut hair. She was walking along a paved path at least one hundred feet inland from the rocky coastline, so the chilled wind caught her by surprise. Still, she welcomed its invigorating caress against her skin.

Two days ago, she had arrived in the small town of Ballyledge on the West Coast of Ireland for a month of…well, she still wasn't quite sure what to call it. Rest and relaxation? Not exactly, given that she had taken an extended leave of absence from Boston General Hospital in order to reevaluate her career as an obstetrician and gynecologist.

It was a chosen profession that meant the world to her. That was until one day seven months ago, when she had lost her own baby daughter as a stillbirth at thirty-two weeks along.

Claire winced as emotions flooded through her, still as raw now as ever. And the words that she had once used to counsel and reassure her own patients who had suffered a miscarriage or stillbirth? Turned inwardly, they brought little comfort as she tried to make sense of her loss.

As a highly regarded double board-certified ob-gyn at the top of her field, Claire knew that it wasn't always possible to pinpoint the reason why a pregnancy ended in miscarriage or stillbirth. An autopsy might have provided some answers, but she hadn't been able to bear to have Ariana's tiny body cut open like that. And she didn't need conclusive evidence to know deep in her heart that her loss had been triggered at least in part by the stress and shock of her then husband Mark walking out on their marriage six months into her pregnancy.

She could deal with the end of her marriage. But the loss of her unborn child? The pain and devastation were so profound that they had extinguished the joy and passion she had once felt for her profession.

You just need some time, everyone had said.

And yet here she was, many months later and seemingly no further along in the healing process. How could she be, when every day in her life as an ob-gyn was a reminder of her loss?

Almost instinctively, Claire touched her lower abdomen, her right hand lingering there for several seconds until she forced herself to lift it away.

Quickening her step along the path, she spotted a smattering of people partaking in various activities on a gently sloping carpet of rich green grass to her left.

It really does look like the color of emeralds, she mused to herself, once again glad that she had chosen Ireland as her getaway destination on not much more than a moment's notice.

It made sense, given that as a proud Irish American, visiting the country had always been on her bucket list. Although she had certainly never imagined that it would be under such trying circumstances.

A smile formed over Claire's lips as she watched a man with two young children—presumably their father—trot across the field as he struggled to control a fluttering kite that was caught in a rip-roaring wind. When he slid on the grass and the kite escaped his grip, twirling upwards until it was little more than a tiny diamond-shaped spot in the sky, she cupped a hand over her mouth as her smile gave way to a chuckle.

It felt good to laugh, to feel the warmth of the sun on her face as the late-morning clouds began to drift further apart. Maybe she'd get through this after all. Maybe she would still find happiness somehow, some way. Perhaps she could take up another area of medicine that wouldn't be a constant reminder of her loss.

Yes, I could do that, she told herself, pushing aside her doubts that she had it in her to start all over again.

Or maybe there was another profession calling to her, outside of the medical field—a previously unfathomable proposition.

She turned to view the coastline, and the small

slice of pale blue water that peeked through the gap between the cliff bluffs and the horizon.

I'll become a painter.

She envisioned herself perched in front of an outdoor easel in a flowing silk scarf and red beret, conveniently ignoring the fact that she could barely draw stick figures.

Or maybe I could try—

Claire's thoughts—and her body—suddenly froze as a woman's agonized shriek reverberated through the air. Catching her breath, she scanned the several small groups of people in the field to her left, her eyes locking in place as they fell upon a woman lying on her back in the grass. A kneeling man hovered over her.

The sight sent a current of ice through Claire's veins. Was he attacking her in broad daylight? And, if so, why was no one rushing to her defense? The kite man was slowly making his way over with his kids, as were several other people who had been walking nearby. But there was no attempt to tackle the man. Something wasn't right.

Wait.

Claire squinted, and then took a deep breath. Even from a distance, there was no mistaking the woman's hugely swollen belly. She was pregnant. And as another guttural scream punctured the otherwise quiet morning, Claire knew one thing for certain.

She's in trouble. I have to help.

It wasn't until she was halfway to the unfolding scene that Claire realized she was running—and fast. It was as if her legs had a mind of their own and her "off" doctor button had been switched back on.

Dropping to her knees beside the woman, she turned to the ashen-faced man who was clutching her hand, his eyes wild with fear. They were both young, quite possibly first-time parents, Claire surmised.

"It's okay," she said breathlessly, her lungs still reeling from her no-holds-barred sprint. "I'm a doctor."

She turned to the woman, equally as pale as her partner, but drenched in sweat, her long dark hair nearly as soaked as if she had just stepped out of the shower. Her light peach cotton maternity top clung to her damp chest. During her quick scan of the woman's body, Claire observed the growing patch of wetness on the inseam of her gray sweatpants. It was all the confirmation she needed that her water had broken.

"I'm Claire," she said, in the soothing tone that was her go-to voice for nervous moms-to-be—and often more so their partners. "What's your name?"

"Margaret," she said in a near-whisper. "And this is my husband, Ted. We were out having a picnic and—" She gasped, grabbing her lower belly, pain gripping her face like a vice.

"Our baby... S-Sam," Ted stuttered. "He's breech."

Two words that cut through the air like a knife.

Claire's throat clamped shut, but he wasn't about to let on that her concern had instantly shifted from medium range to glaring red warning lights.

"We...she has a C-section scheduled in...in..." Ted stammered, unable to say more.

"Three weeks," Margaret managed to say through clenched teeth. "My doctor said this could happen, but I..." She paused to release a barely controlled yelp as another contraction grabbed hold of her.

"But he said it most likely wouldn't," Ted said, finishing his wife's sentence.

Claire tried to piece together the bits of information being volleyed around. "You mean an early labor?"

"Right," Ted replied, nodding vigorously. "He told Margaret to have an overnight bag at the ready, because if her waters broke before the scheduled C-section it would be an emergency situation. Oh, God. What have I done?" Clasping his forehead with jittery hands, he slowly rocked his upper body back and forth. "It was my idea to have a picnic today. I thought the fresh air would do us both some good—"

Claire grabbed Ted's forearm and squeezed it just tightly enough to pull him back into the present. "Ted, I want you to focus, okay? You need to be strong for Margaret. I know you can do this."

He straightened up, the panic in his eyes giving way to resolve. "Right. You're right. Um...um... what can I do?"

Claire glanced at his phone on the ground next to his knee. "Did you call nine-one-one?" It wasn't until she saw the perplexed look on his face that she realized it might not be the same number in Ireland as in the US. "Emergency. Did you call for help?"

"Yes. They said they were sending the nearest ambulance…about ten minutes out."

No sooner had the pronouncement left his mouth than the sound of an approaching siren pierced the air.

Claire turned to Margaret, clasping her free hand with her own. "You're going to be okay, Margaret."

Margaret's gray eyes were clouded with fear. "Sam…"

"Sam is going to be okay, too."

Don't make promises you can't keep.

Reassuring smile still in place, Claire inwardly winced as the obvious crossed her mind. Breech births *were* safe—in a hospital setting. But the chances of them getting to a hospital in time was iffy at best.

"I told you earlier I was a doctor, but I left out an important detail. I'm an ob-gyn, so delivering babies is my specialty."

By now, a small crowd of about a dozen people had gathered around.

"Oh, thank goodness," an older woman said as she puffed out a sigh of relief.

"What are the chances?" a male voice murmured.

What are the chances, indeed? Claire thought.

"Have you delivered breech babies before?" Ted asked anxiously.

"I have. Many times."

Claire's calm voice and reassuring words masked her significant concern. As the ambulance siren grew louder, she forced her mind to filter out the noise so she could be fully present in the moment.

"Did your doctor ever say what type of breech position Sam is in?"

"Um…uh…frank—is that right?" Ted asked, and Margaret replied with a tight squeeze of Claire's hand.

This was slightly better news than a transverse breech, in which the baby was positioned horizontally across the uterus, but dangers still abounded.

"Margaret, I'm just going to feel on your abdomen now," Claire said as she gently pulled her hand away from Margaret's grip. "It's possible Sam has turned on his own, so what I'm trying to determine is the placement of his head."

"I tried everything," Margaret said through gritted teeth as she bit down on her pain. "Acupuncture, chiropractor, tilt exercises…"

"Our doctor tried to turn the baby as well," Ted said. "He wouldn't budge."

It only took several light-pressure pushes on Margaret's abdomen for Claire to confirm that Sam's head was just under her ribcage. *Damn.* She had witnessed many babies flipping into a head-first position in the final days of pregnancy—sometimes just hours before birth—but it was not to be in this instance.

"Is this your first baby?" Claire asked.

Though she was fishing for critical information, she posed the question as casually as possible, so as not to set off further alarms.

"Yes," Margaret replied, smiling weakly as rivulets of sweat rolled down her cheeks.

"We've been over the moon, waiting for Sam to arrive and starting our family," Ted added.

"That's wonderful," Claire said.

She meant it…but the unspoken flipside of this acknowledgement was that a first-time vaginal birth was riskier, especially with a late preterm baby. Sam's small body pushing through the cervix first meant the opening could still be too narrow by the time his head was ready to pass through. If his head were to become stuck before they could reach the hospital, Claire would need to act without delay, flexing and maneuvering it to help bring him into the world as quickly as possible so that he could take that critically important first breath.

Though her intensive training and expert skillset were made for moments like this, Claire couldn't pretend that her nerves weren't on edge. But, as was always the case in a medical emergency, she knew how to fully suppress her fight-or-flight response while staying fully—and calmly—engaged in the moment.

"Thank God! The ambulance is here," a female voice within the small gathering announced.

Claire looked up. The yellow and red box-shaped vehicle slowed to a stop on the road that ran parallel to the walking path, but it was a good five hundred feet or more away. She wondered if it would remain there, which meant the EMTs would have to cover a lot of ground on foot to retrieve Margaret on a stretcher, but seconds later the ambulance pulled off the road and slowly rambled down the green field.

Claire discreetly breathed a sigh of relief—then tensed up as a pair of muscular legs in maroon running shorts appeared just inches away. Her line of vision followed them upwards, settling on a rugged, dark-haired man who looked like he had stepped— or jogged—off the set of a commercial after playing the role of "quintessential Irish hunk."

"I'm a doctor," he said as he kneeled down beside Claire.

Claire did a double-take. He could easily pass for a professional rugby player—but a doctor? It most certainly would not have been her first guess. Still, she was grateful that he had chosen this particular morning and pathway to go for a run. She could use all the help she could get to ensure a safe birth delivery for Margaret and Sam.

"I'm an ob-gyn," she said. "Claire Delaney."

He nodded, thick, tousled hair bobbing as he did. "Kiernan O'Rourke."

"The baby is in a frank breech position," Claire said, her eyes meeting his to silently convey the gravity of the situation. "It's her first pregnancy and she has a C-section scheduled in three weeks."

He pursed his lips together, and Claire felt an unspoken understanding pass between them.

This could be serious. Their lives could be in danger.

"They're probably taking her to West Mercy Hospital in Galway. I'm chief of surgery there." He extracted a phone out of the athletic carry belt around his waist. "I'll call my team to make sure they're on standby."

Claire thought he looked too young to be a chief of surgery, but maybe the climb up the surgical hierarchal ladder proceeded at a quicker pace in Ireland than in the US.

As the ambulance pulled up and came to a stop, the back doors flew open and two EMTs emerged. Kiernan stood up to greet them, pulling a hospital ID badge from the wallet in his belt, which he quietly showed to the pair. Claire observed a subtle shift in the demeanor of both EMTs as they glanced at the badge, then looked up and nodded respectfully.

"I've been in touch with my team at West Mercy and they're awaiting our arrival," Kiernan said.

"Got it," said the young female EMT.

"It's a good thing you came out for a run today, eh?" said the other EMT, a thin man in his fifties with a salt-and-pepper goatee.

"Yes, but she was already in good hands when

I arrived." Kiernan nodded toward Claire. "She's a doctor as well."

"Wow!" the female EMT exclaimed as she and her partner set the stretcher next to Margaret. "That's one heck of a coincidence."

It was all hands on deck as Claire, Kiernan and the EMTs carefully helped Margaret onto the stretcher.

"You're doing great, Margaret," Claire said as she squeezed her hand.

"I don't know if he's going to wait," Margaret said in a near-whisper.

"We're going to get you to the hospital as soon as possible," Claire said.

As the stretcher was loaded into the ambulance and secured into place, both EMTs stepped back outside.

"I'm going to ride in the back with you," Kiernan said, and the male EMT nodded.

"Me, too," Claire quickly added.

The EMT looked at Claire, his expression hesitant. "Are you a doctor at West Mercy as well?"

"No," Claire replied, "I'm a doctor in Boston." She paused, thinking perhaps she shouldn't assume they knew it was a large city on the East Coast of the United States. "It's in—"

"Boston!" The EMT cut her off. "I've got some cousins living there. Nice city. Cold, but nice."

"Go Celtics!" the female EMT said enthusiastically as she referenced the world-famous basketball team that called Boston home.

Her fervent cheer startled Ted, who had been standing several feet away. "Shouldn't I be with my wife?" he asked, his face dazed and his voice equally shaky.

"You can ride with me in the front," the female EMT replied.

He turned to Claire, wide-eyed with worry, and she nodded reassuringly. "It's okay. We'll be watching Margaret closely."

As Ted followed the EMT to the front of the ambulance, her partner gestured to Claire. "I'm sorry, but only authorized medical personnel are allowed to ride in the back."

"Seriously?" Claire asked, unable to hide her displeasure. She looked at Kiernan, waiting for him to overrule the EMT's well-meaning but—in her opinion—misguided decision.

"I'm sorry, but he's right," Kiernan replied, his honey-brown eyes conveying that he wished it were otherwise. "There was an incident a few years back... A man at the scene with a heart attack victim claimed he was a doctor, so they let him on the ambulance while they transported the patient to West Mercy. Turns out he was an imposter."

"That's putting it mildly," the male EMT said as he raised a squirrelly eyebrow. "One of my colleagues was on that run. The guy went berserk inside the ambulance and the patient almost died because of the ruckus."

"That's terrible," Claire conceded. "But I can assure you I'm a real doctor." She paused, her mind racing. "You can look up my name on your phone. I'm an ob-gyn at Boston General."

Kiernan stepped up into the back of the ambulance, turning to face Claire as the male EMT hopped inside and disappeared from view. "I'm sorry," Kiernan said as Margaret screamed through another contraction. "I really am. But we need to leave *now*."

As he shut the left-side ambulance door and started to close the right, Claire's arm shot out, pulling the door open again.

Kiernan's startled look matched her own.

Did I just do that?

She blinked and swallowed hard. Defying orders was so not her thing, but saving lives *was*. And that took precedence over everything.

"Look," she said in a barely controlled low voice. "I get that you're a chief of surgery. But have you ever delivered a frank breech baby? And I don't mean by C-section. Her water broke and she's having contractions. Maybe you'll get to the hospital before the baby enters the birth canal, but you can't guarantee it. And, depending on how he presents, it might take the two of us to turn and maneuver him safely out."

Claire thought she could actually hear the seconds tick by as her stalemate with the handsome chief of surgery continued.

"Well?" she finally asked, rising adrenaline creating an even louder buzz in her head.

* * *

Kiernan stood immobile as he stared at the American doctor who stood just inches away from him. With wavy reddish-brown hair that bounced past her shoulders, porcelain skin and the palest green eyes he had ever seen, she was, without question, one of the most beautiful women he had laid eyes upon. But it wasn't her striking appearance that had frozen him in place. Rather, he had a split-second decision to make—and, in full contrast to his normally resolute, take-charge nature, he wasn't sure what to do.

If he allowed her to accompany this patient and himself to the hospital—potentially assisting in a breech delivery on the way—he would be violating medical emergency transportation laws. And hospital protocol as well. For a chief of surgery, that could have all sorts of repercussions, and none of them good.

Another second passed and Margaret cried out in the throes of a contraction. It was more than enough to jolt him into action.

"Come on," he said, reaching out and pulling Claire up into the ambulance.

She brushed past him, her silky, fruit-scented hair swiping him on the cheek. As the ambulance suddenly took off and began to roll up the grassy field Claire's knees buckled, and she struggled to regain her balance. Kiernan quickly grabbed her arm and pulled her up, her face just inches away from his own.

"Uh…we have a situation here," the EMT announced loudly as Margaret wailed and called out Sam's name.

Kiernan locked eyes with Claire, but only for a second. Rushing over to Margaret, she pulled away from him with such force that it nearly pushed him into the ambulance doors.

"I need gloves," she said to the EMT, her voice growing sharper as she called, "Doctor? I need you over here."

Kiernan was at her side before the words were fully out of her mouth. Snapping on the gloves handed to him by the EMT, he moved in closer and lowered himself while still giving Claire the room she needed to assist with the delivery.

And then he spotted it. Margaret's umbilical cord was protruding, trapped between her pelvic bone and Sam's buttocks, which were lodged in the vaginal opening. He knew that Claire had to find a way to quickly release the pressure on the prolapsed cord, or the baby would be starved of oxygen and blood.

Kiernan took a deep breath and held it in. Standing idly by while another doctor took action was foreign to him, but for once he had to concede that doing so was in the patient's best interest. He barely knew Claire, yet something told him she was an exceptionally gifted ob-gyn. But were they intervening in time? Had the umbilical cord been compressed before they'd loaded Margaret onto the ambulance?

As Claire briefly turned and looked up at him, concern clouding her light green eyes, he couldn't help but think she was silently asking the very same questions.

CHAPTER TWO

"I'LL TAKE FULL RESPONSIBILITY," Kiernan said as the EMT looked wide-eyed at Claire, his lips slightly parted as though he was about to launch a protest.

Eventually he nodded and said, "Just let me know what you need."

"Can you stay close to Margaret, monitor her vitals and coach her breathing?" Claire said.

As the EMT quickly moved toward the front of the stretcher, Claire slid her gloved hand under the baby's partially exposed buttocks, effectively lifting him off the umbilical cord.

She turned to Kiernan, her voice calm and a steely determination in her eyes. "I need you to replace my hand with your own so that I can free his legs."

Kiernan did as instructed, his gloved hand at the ready as Claire slowly slid hers out. "Got it," he said, as he carefully but swiftly lifted the front of Sam's lower torso upwards.

With hands that were considerably larger than Claire's, it was an even tighter squeeze as he concentrated on maintaining the slight yet still sufficient space that would release pressure from the umbilical cord.

With his right shoulder pointed downward at an uncomfortable angle, and Claire pushing up against his stomach as she moved in closer for better positioning, he felt like he was in a medical practitioners' version of the game Twister. A cramp caught him hard in the side, and he cursed under his breath.

Claire looked up at him, her forehead creased as if to say, *What are you bellyaching about?*

"Sorry, I just... I moved the wrong way."

Her face softened slightly, and she nodded before getting back to the task at hand. With her palm pressing down on Sam's lower back, Claire rotated his trunk to the left, then slid her right hand into the vaginal opening, gently looping her fingers around his right leg and pulling it through. Without pause, she moved to the left side and repeated the action with his left leg.

It wasn't until Kiernan saw both legs freed and the rest of Sam's body beginning to inch out that he realized he had been holding his breath the whole time.

"You're doing great, Margaret," Claire called out. Moving her hand next to Kiernan's forearm, she quietly added, "Okay, I'll take it from here."

The exchange of hands was seamless—a feat in itself, given the circumstances, Kiernan thought. He stepped back slightly to give Claire more room. Another contraction sent Sam further out into the world.

"Here come his arms and shoulders," Claire said.

Knowing that they, too, could have become trapped like Sam's legs, Kiernan felt relief that another hurdle had been cleared. All that was left was for his head to emerge.

Clenching his jaw, Kiernan silently encouraged Sam.

You can do it. You're almost there.

It seemed like many minutes passed while Kiernan repeated the silent mantra, though he knew it couldn't have been more than thirty seconds.

From her crouched position, Claire looked up at him. "His head is trapped," she said in a low voice, so as not to alarm Margaret. "I'm going to need a towel…something that I can fold and wrap around his torso."

Kiernan quickly scanned the ambulance interior, then rifled through several supply bins on the left. "Okay, ready when you are," he said, stepping back with a folded towel in his hand.

After placing her right forearm underneath the length of Sam's body, Claire looked up at him. It was the only cue he needed to slide the folded towel between her arm and Sam's torso, lifting him up at an angle that allowed Claire to slide her hand in further.

"I have his jaw…"

Several seconds ticked by. Kiernan knew that she was attempting to place her fingers in Sam's mouth, so that she could better position his head for the next step of the procedure.

"I got it," Claire said, an expression of relief

flooding over her face. She slid her left hand over Sam's back and into the vaginal opening, nodding as she said, "I'm flexing his head downwards. It's coming..."

Without looking up, she instructed Kiernan to push above Margaret's pubic bone with his free hand.

As Sam's head emerged, Kiernan wondered if he had ever witnessed a more wondrous sight. Yes, he was a surgeon. The jack-of-all-trades type, as he was fond of saying whenever anyone asked if he had a specialty. With advanced training and certifications there weren't many surgical areas that he hadn't delved into. Heart bypasses, cancer surgery, joint replacements—he'd done it all. But he had to admit there was something especially poignant about bringing a new life into the world.

Kiernan watched closely, still sending words of encouragement to Sam in his thoughts. The baby boy had officially arrived, but he wasn't fully out of the woods yet. At least not until he took that crucial first breath on his own.

"Betadine," Claire said, her left arm outstretched as Kiernan once again began searching through the supply bins.

"The one on top," the EMT called out.

"Left or right?" Kiernan asked.

"Left."

Kiernan quickly extracted the antibacterial solution and some gauze. Anticipating that Claire would next be asking for clamps and scissors, he grabbed those as well.

Claire wiped the cord with Betadine, then placed two clamps several inches apart. She turned to Kiernan, meeting his eyes. "Do you want to cut the cord?"

She didn't have to ask twice. Snipping the section between the clamps, Kiernan held his own breath as he waited for Sam to take his first. His eyes met Claire's once again, and though no words were said, he knew she was thinking the same dreaded thought.

Had they delivered Sam in time?

"Can I have another towel?" Claire asked urgently.

Kiernan quickly complied, and Claire began vigorously rubbing it over Sam's body.

And then the most glorious sound that Kiernan could ever imagine filled the ambulance.

"I never thought I would be so happy to hear a baby cry," Kiernan said quietly.

A wistful smile crossed Claire's face. "Welcome to the world of obstetrics, where every day is a miracle."

Kiernan couldn't help but notice how she seemed to have momentarily stepped into another time and place, her eyes unblinking, yet focused on nothing in particular, until another surge of sound caused her to snap out of it.

"Sam!" Margaret called out, her voice shaky but unmistakably joyous.

"He's beautiful, Margaret," Claire said, taking the stethoscope that Kiernan had just handed to her.

She placed it over his tiny chest, then looked up at Kiernan and smiled as she nodded. Wrapping Sam in the towel, she lifted him up to Margaret.

"He has a great set of lungs on him, that's for sure," she said as Sam wailed even louder. But once placed in Margaret's arms, he immediately stopped crying.

"He knows where he belongs," the EMT said.

Claire looked up from the mother and baby, nodding to Kiernan with the hint of a smile. It was as if she was silently acknowledging that the two of them had helped make this moment a reality. He smiled and nodded back.

Ten minutes later, the ambulance pulled up to the emergency entrance at West Mercy Hospital. Kiernan hopped out of the vehicle, then turned and offered his hand to Claire as she was about to disembark. She glanced at it before meeting his eyes momentarily. He tried to read the expression on her face. Surprise? Hesitancy? A little of both?

"Thanks," she said, but instead she braced her hand against the open door before stepping carefully out onto the pavement. Given that she hadn't accepted his assistance, he couldn't be sure what she was thanking him for.

As the EMTs rolled the stretcher holding Margaret and Sam toward the entrance, Ted bounded out of the passenger side of the ambulance and ran toward them. Seeing Margaret clutching their tiny newborn son in her arms, he froze in place.

"Oh, my God. Oh, my God. *Oh, my God!*" he exclaimed, his body unlocking as he ran over to the stretcher. "He's beautiful," he said quietly with awe as he beamed down at Sam.

"He certainly is," Margaret said, mustering up the strength to turn her head toward Kiernan and Claire. "And these wonderful doctors saved his life."

Ted turned to Kiernan and Claire. "I don't know how to thank you. This is just…this is the happiest day of my life."

Kiernan smiled and reached out to shake Ted's hand. "Congratulations."

The poor guy is a bundle of nerves, Kiernan thought as Ted continued to shake his hand vigorously, like a wind-up doll with no "off" button.

As smoothly as possible, Kiernan pulled back his hand. He looked over at Claire, knowing that she, too, must be beaming with joy over such a hard-earned happy ending.

Except…she wasn't. Kiernan's own smile faltered as he saw the angst etched on her face. But why? Was it a delayed reaction to the heightened adrenaline and uncertainty that had earlier prevailed, up until the very moment that Sam had been safely delivered? He had seen that sort of thing before with colleagues, after a particularly grueling surgery—even those with miraculous outcomes.

But this felt different.

As though suddenly realizing she was being watched, Claire looked over at him, her eyes meeting his for only a few seconds before she looked away.

Any further contemplation of her strange reaction was cut short by a *swoosh* as the large glass entrance doors swung open. Out strode Lucy, head nurse at West Mercy and Kiernan's right-hand… well, *everything*, given her uncanny ability to stay two steps ahead of his packed daily agenda. And today's unpredictable rollercoaster was no exception.

With a small team of medical professionals behind her, Lucy looked down at the stretcher, her eyes popping open when they landed upon not one, but two occupants.

"We had a bit of an eventful drive on our way over here," Kiernan said, in what he knew could be construed as the understatement of the year.

"I guess so," Lucy said wholeheartedly, a deep smile forming on her lips as she peered down at the new mother and baby. "I would imagine this is one ambulance ride you'll remember for the rest of your life," she said to Margaret.

"I definitely will," Margaret replied with a smile.

"Lucy," Kiernan began, "I'd like you to meet Dr. Claire Delaney. She's visiting from the US and, luckily for Margaret and Sam, she was in the right place at the right time when Margaret went into labor."

"So nice to meet you," Lucy said as she extended her hand.

Claire shook her hand and smiled graciously. "Same here."

Lucy rested both hands on her hips as she turned back to Margaret. "Well, Dr. Preshad is scrubbing in as we speak, expecting that he was going to be performing an emergency C-section. But I'm sure he'll be delighted to know that nature took its course on the way here, and both of you came through with flying colors."

A low rumble of laughter emanated from her team, with Kiernan adding a subdued grin. He wasn't quite at the point where he could look back on the stressful events of the morning and chuckle, but maybe with time. A *lot* of time.

"You've no doubt been through a lot," Lucy continued, "so let's get you inside and settled in."

"Thank you, Doctors," Margaret called out to Kiernan and Claire as two staff members began to wheel the stretcher toward the hospital doors, with Ted close behind.

"Yes, thank you again," Ted called out, before disappearing with the others from view.

Kiernan turned to Claire. "I need to chime in with my huge thanks as well. You truly saved their lives."

"I couldn't have done it without your help."

Though he was tempted to point out that he'd done little more than hand her medical supplies, Kiernan instead smiled and accepted the compliment. "I'm just glad we were both at the right place, at the right time."

"Me too."

"Say, while you're here, I'd love to show you around our new neonatal wing. It's scheduled to be fully up and running in another month. It might not have all the bells and whistles that you're used to at a big-city hospital like Boston General, but it's close. In fact, one of our longer-range goals is to offer cutting-edge neonatal care and the latest treatment options that aren't widely available. And I don't just mean for this region, but for the entire country."

Claire smiled.

Finally, Kiernan thought.

"That's sounds wonderful. And certainly ambitious." She paused, and there was a distinct look of pain in her eyes. "But I have to leave now."

It was not the answer Kiernan had expected, and he wasn't prepared to reply. Finally, he managed to utter, "Oh?"

"Yes, sorry. I have to…there's…um… I have to be somewhere."

Kiernan studied the stunning but increasingly mysterious woman before him. He didn't believe for a second that she had to be somewhere else. An incredibly talented doctor? Yes. But a convincing actress? Not so much.

"Well, I'm not sure how long you're staying in Ireland, but I'd be happy to give you a tour another time."

Kiernan creased his brow as he waited for her reply.

Why is she looking at me like I'm asking her to tour a room full of rattlesnakes and tarantulas?

"That's nice of you to offer. But I'm not sure I'll have time while I'm here."

"I understand," Kiernan said, although nothing could be further from the truth. "No problem."

Claire slid her phone from the back pocket of her jeans and tapped on the screen. "I did a search before coming here about whether there are Ubers in Ireland…" She looked up at Kiernan. "The answer was yes, but they're actual taxis—not drivers in their personal cars. Kind of defeats the purpose of an Uber," she added with a nervous laugh.

"Look, I'm heading back to Ballyledge myself. Why don't you ride with me? It's the least I can do after you saved the day like you did. The hospital has a small fleet of cars that are used for patient transport. I'll have one of my staff take us back."

Claire's smile vanished faster than the flipping of a light switch. She looked down at her phone. "Actually, it looks like I have a ride that's two minutes out."

Kiernan forced a smile. There was no point suggesting that she cancel the taxi and ride back with him instead. For whatever reason—despite what he felt had been a connection between them as they'd worked together to save Margaret and Sam—she wanted nothing more to do with him.

"That was fast," Claire said just over a minute and a half later as she waved to a taxi heading toward them. As the taxi came to a stop, she turned to

Kiernan. "It was nice meeting you. And thank you for helping me with the delivery. I really couldn't have done it without you."

Kiernan was about to insist otherwise, but stopped himself. She was merely trying to be polite, so no need to point out that he'd done little more than hold a folded towel and grab some supplies. Not when she had made it clear that she wanted to leave as soon as possible.

Opening the taxi passenger door, he waited for her to be seated before saying, "Take care of yourself. And enjoy your stay in Ireland."

Another skittish smile. "I will. Thank you."

As Kiernan watched the taxi drive away, he heard footsteps approach from behind. Dr. Sebastian Kincaid, an anesthesiologist and one of Kiernan's best friends since medical school, swaggered up to him.

"*Who* was *that*?"

Kiernan rolled his eyes—a reaction he didn't in the least bit bother to hide from Sebastian. Known as a real-life Dr. McDreamy by half of the female staff at West Mercy who regularly ogled him for his perpetually tanned skin, thick sandy-blonde hair and gym-aficionado physique, he had also earned the moniker of Dr. McDouchebag from the other half who'd had the misfortune of actually dating him at one time or another.

"That's Claire Delaney. She's an American doctor who happened to be walking nearby when the patient we just brought in went into labor. And a breech presentation, no less. She was pretty amazing delivering the baby. I'll tell you that."

"Pretty amazing, huh? I'm sure she was," Sebastian noted with his usual lack of subtlety. A pained grunt followed as Kiernan elbowed him sharply in the ribs. "What's that for?"

Kiernan grinned. "For you being you."

Sebastian straightened himself up, still rubbing his side. "So, how long is she here for?"

"I have no idea."

"Seriously? You didn't get her number or anything? What—are you losing your touch?"

Kiernan sighed exasperatedly as he raised an eyebrow. "Yes, well… I decided to hold off hitting on her while she was delivering a breech baby in the back of a bumpy ambulance." He paused for full dramatic effect. "I'm silly like that."

Sebastian shook his head, but with a smirk and a twinkle in his eyes. "You know, I really thought once you made chief of surgery you'd finally loosen up and realize that there's more to life than work."

"And why would you think that?"

"You're at the top of the food chain now. Which means it's time to enjoy some of the fruits of your labor. So to speak."

As Sebastian winked and wiggled his eyebrows, Kiernan reluctantly grinned.

"You've got the goods, mate," Sebastian continued. "You just need to show more of your authentic self, that's all."

Kiernan was beginning to lose patience. Fast. *"What?"*

"Remember that speaker we had here a few months ago, who talked about how to avoid career burnout? She mentioned the importance of bringing our authentic selves to work. You know—being real human beings and not just the series of medical credentials after our names. No one—besides myself, of course—feels like they really know you. That's all. A little banter here and there, some joking around, sharing your weekend plans—or at least pretending you have some… Things like that could go a long way."

Kiernan stared at him hard. "Remind me again why we're friends?"

Sebastian smiled, revealing teeth so white that Kiernan wondered if he should don sunglasses.

"Because you need me. I'm the best wingman you'll ever have—even though you refuse to take advantage of my services."

"I'm head of the surgery department. I see people whose lives are at stake, day in and day out. I don't have time to mollycoddle my colleagues."

Sebastian stared at him, his mouth twisted to one side. "Right. If you say so," he finally said, this time slapping Kiernan on the other shoulder. He looked at his watch. "Well, I'm off to prep for a gallbladder removal."

He took a few steps in the direction of the hospital entrance, and then he stopped and swiveled around.

"And by the way... No one says 'mollycoddle' anymore. Other than time travelers from the nineteenth century."

He flashed a smile and gave a thumbs-up before turning on his heels and continuing on his way.

Kiernan sighed, then shook his head and managed a weary smile.

Bring your authentic self to work. Who comes up with this stuff, anyway?

And yet...

His thoughts turned to Claire, and the incredibly intense turn of events that had brought them so briefly together. Two complete strangers, working in tandem to save the lives of a mother and her newborn baby.

It doesn't get any more real than that, he thought.

But as he replayed their parting of ways in his mind, he was faced with another reality, and this one left a sting in its wake.

She couldn't get away from me fast enough.

Claire watched silently from the back passenger window of the taxi as rolling green fields, stone walls and the occasional grazing sheep whizzed past. Ten minutes ago they had left the city limits of Galway, and viewing the quiet countryside was like a calming elixir for her soul. Which was something she certainly needed right now.

Another patchwork of green fields, this time grazing goats, and Claire turned away from the window, leaning back against the headrest. She closed her eyes and breathed in deeply, feeling as though it was her first full breath since the moment she had knelt down on the ground beside Margaret.

Slowly, she shook her head. Was the universe trying to mess with her mind? She had come to Ireland for a reprieve from her life as a baby doctor, and only days in she'd been thrown back into it in the most unexpected and harrowing way.

Dabbing at her moist eyes with the sleeve of her cardigan, she caught the driver glancing at her through the rearview mirror. She hoped he would look away, and was relieved when he finally did.

It will pass, she told herself.

Not the pain that she still felt from losing Ariana, but the tears that flowed every time a situation triggered her emotions into overdrive.

Still… As she thought of the exhausted but overjoyed Margaret, holding tiny Sam in her arms, she couldn't help but think that maybe the universe knew what it was doing after all. Yes, a yet to be fully healed wound in her heart had been tugged open. But now there was a very happy new mom and a healthy baby boy who might not have had the same outcome if it hadn't been for her and a chief of surgery who had also been in the right place at the right time.

Her mind wandered again. And this time she didn't call it back. Not when it had settled upon a handsome doctor with a rugged build and kind brown eyes. Kiernan O'Rourke. Now, *that* was an Irish name, she mused to herself. Her emerging smile halted as she thought about how earlier she had cut him off at the knees. He was just trying to be friendly by offering a hospital tour, one doctor to another, and she had abruptly declined.

I have to be somewhere.

She rolled her eyes at what must have come across as the lamest excuse ever.

In another day or two he'll forget all about it, Claire told herself.

At least that was what she hoped. The last thing she would ever want to do was hurt another person's feelings. And something told her that was especially true of the attractive Irish doctor who had just helped her bring a new life into the world.

CHAPTER THREE

CLAIRE PLOPPED DOWN on the small couch with its lopsided cushions in her quaint two-room rental cottage. It was early Tuesday evening, three days since that whirlwind of medical drama had left her spinning on every level.

She had arrived in Ireland with no game plan other than to engage in some much-needed soul-searching. But, even so, she recognized that her tendency to withdraw from others when dealing with a personal issue was not doing her any favors right now. Perhaps it was time to switch things up. No one had to know the real reason she was in Ireland for an extended stay. So why not seek out some group activities…like a guided tour of castles?

Great idea, she thought as she proceeded to search for local attractions on her phone.

A notification icon popped up on her screen and she stared at it for several seconds. If there was one sound piece of advice that had come out of her therapy sessions, it was to stay off social media as much as possible. The algorithms had a way of knowing what was on your mind and only feeding you more of it—whether "it" was something good or bad. She had long ago removed her ex-husband

Mark from any social media friends list but, both being doctors, they had so many mutual acquaintances in the medical world that she couldn't be certain he wouldn't pop up in someone else's post when least expected.

Still, what was the harm in tapping on one update? Maybe it would be a fun kitten or puppy video—always guaranteed to bring a smile.

She opened the notification…and her heart stopped.

Staring back at her was a photo of Mark, cradling an infant in his arms. *Daddy celebrates three months of diaper duty and butterfly kisses with his little girl!* the caption read, followed by hearts and smiles emojis.

Furiously scanning the post, Claire quickly discovered it had originated on the page of Christine White, a physician assistant at Mark's internal medicine practice. Just as she had been warned, Christine's post had found its way onto her phone as a "people you may know" notification.

She closed her eyes, somehow managing to do the math in her head that confirmed Christine had been pregnant with Mark's child when he had walked out on her and Ariana. She shouldn't be surprised. She *wasn't* surprised. And yet the revelation still cut like a knife.

The blade went even deeper as she recalled how Mark had been contacted by the hospital when she was about to have labor induced for the stillbirth of Ariana. He couldn't be bothered to come. The depths of his cold indifference to his own flesh and blood were almost inconceivable…but he had started a new family, and had already rendered her and Ariana inconsequential.

A few more moments of pained disbelief and then Claire shook her head, as though she could physically dislodge all of the distressing thoughts.

Time to pull yourself up by the bootstraps, she instructed herself.

She hadn't traveled three thousand miles just to sit in a small cottage and brood, now, had she? Well, maybe she had, but that was about to change.

When in Rome…

Okay, she was in Ballyledge, which most certainly wasn't Rome, but it had more than its share of charm and possibilities.

Rising from the couch and walking several steps to a side window, she looked out onto the purplish-orange sky as dusk set in. Her mind flashed back to a cute little pub that had caught her eye the previous day, while she'd been picking up groceries in the village. Overlooking the water, and with an outdoor terrace softly lit by string lights, it had just the right vibe to help ease her out of her slump. Or so she hoped.

Before she had a chance to talk herself out of her sudden plan, Claire headed to the bathroom to brush her hair, put on some clear lip gloss, then stare in the mirror as she declared, "You. Can. Do. This."

Twenty minutes later she was seated at a small

wooden table on the outside terrace of Gilroy's Pub, watching the rising moon cast an ethereal glow over the inland bay. The low hum of conversation around her was just enough of a reminder that she was not alone. But that all changed in an instant as a loud, rambunctious group of men tumbled onto the terrace.

I might as well be in an American sports bar, Claire thought as she turned to look at the sweaty, disheveled men.

Their blue and white shorts and matching shirts were streaked with dirt and mud, and their metal-cleated shoes sounded like a herd of horses galloping to the barn for their oats. Not exactly the ambiance she was expecting at the pub, but then again, was it really so bad to witness a group of guys having some rabble-rousing fun?

Nope, Claire concluded, but she still turned away and refocused her gaze on the shimmering bay.

"Dr. Delaney?"

Claire swung her head around, then did a double-take as her eyes landed on Dr. Kiernan O'Rourke.

"I thought that was you," he said, briefly glancing at the chair across from her.

It was more than enough of a cue for her to ask him to have a seat. As he pulled up the chair, Claire's mouth was still slightly agape. Whether it was from the overall surprise of seeing him again, or the fact that West Mercy's chief of surgery was now sitting across from her with a patch of dirt caked on one cheek and a nasty scratch etched across the other, she couldn't be sure.

"This is quite the surprise, Dr. O— Mr. O'Rourke." Suddenly remembering that Irish surgeons use honorific titles, Claire caught herself just in time.

"Please, call me Kiernan. With all we went through the other day, at the very least we should be on a first-name basis."

Claire dipped her head as she smiled, then added, "Claire. Nice to meet you—again." After a slight pause, she shook her head and laughed quietly.

Kiernan cocked his head. "I'd ask if you were laughing *with* me, except I haven't told a joke."

"I'm sorry. It's just that… Well, the first time I saw you, I thought you looked like a professional rugby player."

"Ahh." Kiernan appeared almost relieved. "And then you discovered I'm just the boring chief of surgery at West Mercy Hospital."

Claire smirked. "No—it's not like that at all. More like, what are the chances that I'd see you again and you really *do* play rugby. At least I think that's a rugby uniform you're wearing. Or is it soccer?" She tapped her hand to her mouth. "Oops, I mean football."

"You saved yourself just in time," Kiernan joked. "In fact, I'm not sure if the word 'soccer' is officially banned from Ireland, but it should be."

Claire chuckled. "Point taken."

"But, yes, I play in a local rugby league. We usually have a match every Tuesday night from spring to late autumn."

"So you live in the area?"

"I do. I have a house about five miles from here. Up on a high bluff and overlooking the ocean— just in case I ever decide to take up cliff-diving in the spare time that I don't have." He paused. "You look surprised."

"That you might take up cliff-diving?" Claire replied, gamely playing along.

He grinned. "That I live in town."

"I guess I am...sort of. Working at the hospital in Galway—I would have figured you lived in the city."

Kiernan nodded his head from side to side, as though weighing her observation, his thick dark hair bobbing back and forth in unison. "That's a reasonable assumption. And I did live there for a few years."

"Oh?"

"I came back because I grew up in Ballyledge, and I may be biased, but I don't think there are many more pristine spots in the country."

"The scenery is breathtaking, that's for sure," Claire agreed.

"Plus, it helps keep me grounded. I'm sure I don't have to tell you that working in a hospital—especially on difficult cases when lives are in the balance—is like a constant adrenaline rush that can be hard to come down from. But here..." he nodded toward the water "...the sound of the waves crashing up against the rocks, with no one around other than some egrets and a few seals—it helps put things in perspective."

Claire gestured appreciatively. "Poetically said."

Kiernan took a sizeable sip of beer. "I kind of surprised myself with that one." As Claire laughed, he added, "Okay, now it's your turn."

Claire's laughter quickly petered out. "My turn?" she asked, wide-eyed. Her mind raced as she tried to think of what to say.

Keep it light. And happy. And...

"I didn't mean to put you on the spot," Kiernan said, viewing her through perplexed eyes.

It took some effort, but Claire found her smile once more. "No—that's fine. I was just trying to think of something that might be remotely interesting."

Kiernan raised an eyebrow, his expression equal parts surprised and amused. "I just spent two hours on a muddy field listening to nothing but grunts, burps and the splat of projectile spits. So trust me when I say *anything* you'd like to share about yourself right now will be infinitely more fascinating by comparison."

Claire snickered, feeling her guard drop a notch, not just emotionally, but physically as well. The release of tension in her neck and shoulders was a welcome respite. "Okay, well... I always wanted to visit Ireland, and here I am." She paused, debating whether to go one step further. "For a month."

Slow down there, girl, she chided herself inwardly.

"Now, see? *That* was interesting." Kiernan studied her closely, as if trying to discern more through sheer will.

Good luck with that, she thought.

"Did you come here with others?"

As Claire shook her head, she could almost see the intrigue growing in his eyes.

"Did you come here to visit someone, then?"

"Nope."

Kiernan sat back in his chair, crossing his arms and grinning at the same time, as though relishing the challenge before him. "So, why Ireland?"

"It's an Irish American thing, I guess. We all want to visit the motherland, so to speak, at some point in our lives."

"Delaney," Kiernan said with a nod. "Of course. And the hospital is okay with you being away for a whole month?"

Claire swallowed hard, her heart momentarily surging in her chest before quieting down. She needed to steer the conversation away from her career—which ultimately led back to babies—and fast.

"Boston General's good about encouraging us to take time off as needed."

"I see. That's great." He paused, another grin emerging. "I feel like I'm on one of those game shows where I'm trying to guess someone's back story with limited clues."

Claire smirked, realizing she was about to let her guard down a teeny-weeny bit more, but was surprisingly okay with that. "Go ahead—give it your best shot."

"All right, then." Kiernan glanced down at her unadorned wedding ring finger, then back up at her, his warm brown eyes latching onto her own. "You're here alone, so either there's no husband or kids at home, or you decided you needed a bit of a break from them, too."

Her smile faltered for a fraction of a second, but she managed to recover it. "No husband or kids."

He cocked his head to the side. "Hmm…the plot thickens. So you came here in the hopes of meeting some strapping Irishman who looks like he stepped off the set of a commercial?"

Claire had just taken a sip of wine, and in short order choked on it as Kiernan unknowingly voiced her silent assessment of him at their first meeting.

Kiernan chuckled. "I think I'm on to something. Ten points for contestant number three."

Claire waved him away as she coughed some more. "I just swallowed the wrong way, that's all."

"Right…" he said, clearly unconvinced.

She laughed, perplexed at the high level of comfort she felt around Kiernan, but determined to go with the flow.

"Okay," Kiernan began. "I've put you on the hot seat long enough. Now it's your turn to ask me a question."

Claire ran her index finger over the rim of her

wine glass as she stalled for time. So many possible questions, but best to keep it light. "Did the hospital make you take out an insurance policy on your hands when they heard you were playing a rough contact sport on the side?"

Kiernan laughed, then held up his hands in mock examination. Claire felt a swish of butterflies in her stomach as she admired their obvious strength and masculinity. Not what she would normally picture as "surgeon's hands," but she certainly had no complaints about the view.

"No, but they did suggest I trade in rugby for badminton."

Claire chuckled. "Somehow I can't picture you daintily prancing up to a badminton net."

Kiernan laughed heartily. "You got that right."

"Let's see… You live high up on a bluff, but no cliff-diving as of yet?"

"Correct. I'm waiting for the cliffs to shrink to the size of ant hills."

Claire grinned. "Do you live alone?"

"I do."

"Is that a good thing or a bad thing?"

Kiernan teetered his head back and forth, as though weighing his answer. "I would say it's a good thing."

"Just a man in his castle?"

Kiernan looked amused. "Something like that."

"So, no wife and kids in your future, or you just haven't met the right woman?"

Careful, Claire…

"I suppose the latter—although some might say I'm married to my profession."

There were so many possible replies to that—some humorous, some cutting—but Claire chose instead to safely change the subject. Except that no alternative subject immediately came to mind.

Keep it happy, she reminded herself once again. *Nothing too deep...*

"Which is probably just as well," he went on. "Since I don't foresee any children in my future."

It took a few moments for Claire to realize that her face must have frozen into a mask of shock. How else to explain why Kiernan's smile had instantly faded, and his forehead visibly tensed as he attempted to explain himself further.

"I only mention that because you asked."

"Yes… Right… Not everyone wants kids. Nor should everyone have them, based on some of the horrors I've seen as a doctor. And you, too, I'm sure."

"Unfortunately, yes. But for me personally, it's more like I've learned from the mistakes of my own father. He was a surgeon, too. A *brilliant* surgeon, I should add. He helped pioneer some of the first organ laparoscopic surgeries. But he was a lousy father. I know it sounds crass to say that about one's own parent, but he'd probably be the first to admit it himself if he were still here."

"He's passed away?" Claire asked as delicately as possible, still reeling from Kiernan's unexpected revelation, but doing her best to hide that fact.

Kiernan nodded. "Three years ago. In the last five years of his life, we actually forged some semblance of a relationship. Although it was more like a friendship based on a shared interest in medicine rather than a father-and-son kind of thing. He did finally acknowledge that he'd been an absentee father for most of my life. I think that's why he felt it important to advise me not to have kids if I truly wanted to be the best surgeon I could possibly be."

"Hmm... That's interesting."

Kiernan cocked his head slightly to one side, a look of curiosity in his eyes. "What's interesting?"

"That instead of telling you not to make the mistake of putting career over family, he essentially told you the opposite."

Kiernan was silent for a moment. "I never really looked at it like that, but I suppose you're right."

"And your mom?"

Kiernan's face brightened. "My mum is doing great. She lives about a half-hour from here in an independent living community. I don't think she realized how much she was living in my dad's shadow until he passed away. Now, she's made new friends, has taken up gardening as a hobby, and to be honest, I don't think I've ever seen her happier."

"Well, I've obviously never met your mom, but I'm glad to hear that."

She had never met his father, either, but she sure was getting a picture of an overbearing man who may have been a genius with a scalpel, but couldn't quite cut it as a father or a husband.

"And what about your family?" Kiernan asked.

"I lost my dad, too, also three years ago. We were very close, so it was hard. Still is, some days. My mom lives in one of those nice little New England towns outside of Boston. You know—the kind that have old historical houses with placards that say, *Paul Revere rode past here to warn colonists about approaching British troops.*"

That observation elicited a chuckle from Kiernan, prompting Claire to laugh as well.

"I have a younger brother who works in finance and lives in New York, still doing the bachelor thing despite my mom's matchmaking attempts. And I have a sister, Grace, who works in real estate and is two years older than me. She moved to Pennsylvania recently, when my brother-in-law relocated for a job promotion, and she has two young sons. They're great kids and I love being an aunt."

Kiernan smiled. "Well, I think I know you better now than I know most of my colleagues."

Was he joking? Claire couldn't be sure. She had certainly known her share of doctors who were all business while on duty, but Kiernan didn't strike her as the uptight, humorless type. Then again, they weren't in a hospital environment at the moment. Perhaps he felt the need to maintain a measure of personal detachment from his colleagues as chief of surgery—and, given the monumental responsibility of the role, that was understandable.

But before she could contemplate things further, Kiernan's rugby teammates came barreling over, surrounding their table and kicking up an aromatic cloud of sweat, dirt and beer.

"Is he bothering you?" a gargantuan man with hands the size of baseball mitts slurred, as he tried to focus through red-tinged eyes.

"Not at all," Claire replied with a wink in Kiernan's direction.

"He's a great catch, this one, you know," another teammate said with a wallop on Kiernan's back that nearly shook the table. "He's a surgery bigwig. Which is good—because he'd never make it as a professional rugby player."

As the teammate topped off this observation with a hard knock of his knuckles on Kiernan's skull, Claire winced. "Oh…careful! That had to hurt."

Kiernan chuckled—but not before slugging his buddy hard in the thigh from where he sat.

"Eh… I've been punched harder by my ninety-year-old grandmother," the teammate said, though his bulging eyes and creased forehead suggested otherwise.

Kiernan backed up his chair a bit. "Well, I'd love to continue this scintillating conversation with you brutes, but…*no.* You can leave now."

He pointed to the terrace bar—not that they needed directions on how to return to their temporary watering hole.

After some good-natured grumblings and a few rounds of friendly slaps and punches, the group retreated to the other side of the pub.

"Wow!" Claire exclaimed, before breaking into laughter.

"Not the most subtle bunch, huh?" Kiernan replied as he shook his head, a half-smile on his lips.

"Last orders!" the bartender boomed from behind the counter.

Claire glanced at her watch. "Geez, that went by fast."

"Can I get you another glass of wine?" Kiernan asked as he nodded toward her empty glass.

The word "sure" was about to roll off her lips. And then…reality set in, bringing with it a slew of blinking red caution lights. She would be leaving Ireland in less than a month.

He doesn't want kids!

Even though she knew he was simply being polite in asking if she wanted a drink at last call, she couldn't deny that she felt a growing attraction to him. So why tempt herself with a situation that could never be? She might be putting the cart before the horse, but it was for her own good. She had come to Ireland to find clarity and to heal—not to muddy the waters with a strong but dead-end attraction.

Claire slowly pushed back her chair and stood up. "Thanks, but I think I'm going to head back to my cottage now. I must still be grappling with some jet lag, because I feel like it's three in the morning!"

Really, Claire, another lame excuse?

She could tell by his pinched expression that Kiernan wasn't buying her explanation for a second. And the fact that this pinched face was still one of the most handsome she had ever encountered… Well, that was reason alone to conclude that she was doing the right thing.

Kiernan stood up from his chair. "Did you walk here?"

"I did. It only took me fifteen minutes. I'm staying at one of the pink cottages about a mile that way," she said, pointing west.

"Ah, the pink cottages—which used to be white, by the way," Kiernan noted. "There's a rumor that the owner refurbished them while on an acid trip, but you didn't hear that from me."

Claire snickered. "I did wonder about the color… not going to lie. But they're cute, and it's sort of the perfect little home-away-from-home while I'm here."

"Well, let me at least walk you back."

Claire forced a smile to mask the discomfort that was expanding inside. "I'm fine, really. It's not like walking back through some dark Boston alley. In fact, I went for a walk last night along the pier and it was really quite beautiful." She looked up at the sky. "The moon and stars were out in full force, just like tonight."

Kiernan watched her silently for several moments, his lips pressed tightly together. Finally, he nodded and managed a smile. "Well, if you get bored and want someone to talk to over the next few weeks I'm here every Tuesday evening with my fellow louts. I'm occasionally here on late Sunday afternoons, too. There's a team practice that I join when I can, and we usually wind down afterwards with a pint or two."

"I'll keep that in mind," Claire said, truly appreciative of his offer.

Kiernan's lips curved into a slight grin. "Oh— and one more thing. If you decide to hit up the usual tourist spots, you might want to spray the Blarney Stone with a strong antiseptic before kissing it. Just saying…"

Claire chuckled quietly. "That's good advice."

"By the way, how are you getting around? Do you have a car?"

"I rented a Mini. A little red one. Goes perfectly with the pink house."

Kiernan smiled and nodded. "Good choice. Well, you take care."

"You, too."

As Claire walked past him, unable to fully divert her eyes away from his muscular body as it pressed against his taut athletic shirt, it was as if something grabbed hard at her stomach.

Once outside, she took a deep breath and allowed the cool night air to seep into her lungs. For a split second she questioned her decision to close the door—no, make that *slam* the door—on any further interaction with Kiernan. But she had no choice. She had come to Ireland to make a difficult decision that could potentially alter the course of her life from hereon in. The last thing she needed was to tempt another complication that would only create more heartache. She had had enough of that for a lifetime already.

Kiernan walked into the still-dark kitchen of his home and tossed his keys onto the counter. Switching on the light, he felt as though he could hear the emptiness that surrounded him. There were plenty of inanimate objects in view, of course, and some, like the refrigerator, emitted a low-level hum that could pass for a sign of life, albeit an electronic one.

But no human voices. No greeting from a loving partner, no joyful screeches of an excited child.

Not even a bark or a meow.

And although he had once toyed with the idea of getting a couple of goldfish, even that had fallen by the wayside when he'd considered the possibility that his fairly frequent one, two or even three-nighters at the hospital meant potentially coming home to fish that were floating belly-up in a tank.

The irony that he could save lives in the direst of situations as a surgeon but couldn't sustain a pet goldfish—or even a companion plant—was not lost on Kiernan.

He grimaced as he opened a bottle of electrolyte-infused water, staring blankly at the bland, cream-colored wall as he took several long sips. He was used to being met by silence upon returning home—found comfort in it, actually—but tonight something felt different.

He wondered if his reaction had been spawned

by the look on Claire's face when he had mentioned his intention to live a child-free life. She had seemed surprised by his revelation, if not momentarily disturbed, but should she have been? How could any doctor at the top of their game feel differently?

He placed the bottle on the counter and sighed, knowing well the answer to his own question.

Because not every doctor had a father like you.

Which, depending on how he looked at it, was both a blessing and a curse.

The blessing was that he'd inherited his father's innate ability to excel as a surgeon—a combination of empirical knowledge, think-outside-the-box innovation and exceptional dexterity that had turned his hands into lifesaving instruments.

The curse was…well, it was the very same thing. Because—just like his father—he had an unrelenting desire to constantly improve. And continually expanding his skillset and saving more lives didn't just happen on its own. It required devotion to a singular purpose. Day in and day out. *Year* in and *year* out.

His father had made the mistake of thinking that if he cut back from one hundred percent devotion to his career to ninety-five percent, and directed the remaining five percent to his family, it would be enough. How wrong he had been. Those sparse breadcrumbs had been no substitute for his presence at the primary school play or the secondary school rugby game.

Even career advice had been more aptly dispensed by the school's advisor than his own father. When Kiernan had told his father that he was applying to the School of Medicine at Trinity College—his father's alma mater—the detached reply had been: "Don't expect to coast on my coattails if you get in." Not *I'm so proud of you* or *You'll make a great surgeon*.

His dad had relayed one more nugget of advice that Kiernan had taken to heart, though: "You'd better not entertain trying out for the Trinity rugby team if you do get in. You need to devote one thousand percent to your studies, otherwise you'll never make it."

Kiernan smiled wistfully as he recalled one of his first actions upon starting his freshers year. Not only had he tried out for Trinity's football team, but he'd been the star inside center up until graduation. Had it been a safe act of rebellion on his part? Perhaps. But he couldn't have rebelled by choosing an alternative profession—that would have only hurt him, not his dad.

He was doing what he was meant to do. And he had learned from his father's mistakes. He would forgo having a family of his own not because he was cold inside, or because he had no affinity for children, but because he *did*. And he would never want them to suffer the loneliness and insecurity that he had felt as a young boy, growing up with a father who was a parent in name only.

Kiernan shuddered as he pulled himself back to

the present. That was then, and this was now. Yes, there had been more than a few romantic relationships that had skidded to a halt once the topic of children had been broached, but better to know upfront that his priorities were a deal-breaker for someone. The simple fact was that most women wanted a family of their own—and he would never want to deny them that source of joy and fulfillment.

Perhaps he was destined to sail through life unattached, and he was okay with that. Well, it was more like he had come to accept that this was his fate. It was a choice he'd made knowingly and willingly—career over commitment—and he had yet to regret his decision.

His thoughts turned to Claire, her face coming into sharp focus in his mind. The pale but piercing green eyes, the full, pillowy lips and rich chestnut hair. What was her real story, anyway? Why was she taking a whole month off from her critical role as an ob-gyn at a major Boston hospital? Why had she come to Ireland all alone? Was it some sort of American thing? She certainly didn't strike him as the flighty type—quite the opposite, actually—but something just didn't add up.

Not that he would ever get answers to his questions. Unless Claire decided to deliberately show up at the pub when he was there—and he highly doubted she would—he was never going to see her again. She had disappeared into the darkness of the night like Cinderella, leaving him with no means to contact her. Instead of a glass slipper, he needed…what? A hospital-grade clog to try and track her down?

Perhaps it was just as well, Kiernan thought. Something told him he could fall hard for the intriguing American doctor who had suddenly appeared in his life. And that, quite simply, did not fit in with his ultimate plan.

CHAPTER FOUR

"THERE YOU ARE," Lucy said to Kiernan as he looked up from his tablet.

Though he would admit it to no one, he sometimes longed for the days—not so far in the past—when he could rifle through physical charts rather than be tapping ad nauseam on a digital screen.

"What is it with this thing?" Kiernan said impatiently as he pressed on "lab results" and up popped a list of the patient's current medications instead. "Are my fingers too fat or something?"

Lucy twisted her mouth to one side. "No, I'm sure it's just that the tabs are too small."

Placing the tablet onto the nurses' station counter with an exasperated sigh, he turned to Lucy. "Nice try."

"I do my best."

"Were you looking for me?"

"I was. It's about Jan Reddy—her ultrasound last week showed fetal spina bifida."

"Yes…right. I haven't met with her personally, but her case came up in the weekly staff meeting."

Lucy nodded. "She's here for more tests this morning, and I was wondering if maybe you'd be able to talk to her. She's having a hard time dealing with the diagnosis, especially since her surgery options are still up in the air."

"Of course. I'll swing by and see her. I thought we had our scheduling staff looking into fetal surgery availability at other hospitals?"

"They are, but no luck as of yet."

Kiernan grimaced. It was not the news he wanted to hear. Fetal surgery for spina bifida offered hope for babies that were developing in the womb with an open gap in their spinal cord. But it was an extremely complex surgery that only certain hospitals were equipped to offer, and West Mercy wasn't one of them.

Kiernan hoped that this would change once the new neonatal wing was up and running, but even then it would most likely be some way down the road. It took a very gifted surgeon to perform this delicate operation, and although he had many exceptional surgeons on his staff, none were trained in this type of procedure. All of which meant Jan would have to find another hospital that could schedule the surgery in time, and even if that was possible it would mean significant personal expense and possibly traveling away from her two young children.

"Okay, keep me posted. I'll probably touch base with Dr. Fleming first," he said, referring to Jan's obstetrician, "but I'll check in on Jan right after."

"Great, thanks," Lucy replied. She nodded toward the tablet on the counter. "Don't forget to take your friend with you on your travels. As of last count, it's been brought to a nurses' station on every floor and designated as 'lost' no less than a dozen times."

Kiernan shot an annoyed glance at the device. "Yeah, well... I guess subconsciously I keep hoping that it won't find its way back to me."

Lucy smirked. "Progress, Mr. O'Rourke. It's a good thing, I promise."

Once Lucy had departed, Kiernan took a moment to organize his thoughts. Per usual, he had a busy day ahead, but he preferred to map it out in his mind rather than record it on the tablet.

"Hey, hey, hey, my man!" Sebastian exclaimed as he suddenly inserted himself in front of Kiernan like a photo-bombing squirrel.

"Not you again," Kiernan replied with a mixture of annoyance and friendly affection.

"Listen, that hot American doctor from the other day... I got the goods on her."

Now *this* had Kiernan's attention. "What do you mean?"

"I discovered she's got quite the resume back at Boston General."

Kiernan's voice grew sharper. "And how exactly did you find this out?"

Sebastian let loose with a crocodile smile. "Simple. You told me her name..." The smile grew impossibly wider. "And Google is my friend."

Kiernan slid the tablet off the counter and tucked it under his arm. "Good, because you don't have any others."

Like all of Kiernan's pretend insults, this one rolled off Sebastian like water off a duck. "My, my, we're touchy today. I was certain you'd want to know that she's considered an expert in high-risk pregnancies and cutting-edge fetal surgery. And she's got quite the list of awards and distinctions."

"I'm not surprised," Kiernan said. "I saw first-hand what she's capable of."

Sebastian ran his fingers through his perfectly coiffed hair, then leaned his elbow on the counter. "You think she's still in the area? I bet I could find out where she's staying. I've never played tour guide before, but for her I'd make an exception."

Kiernan viewed him through narrowed eyes. "And I've never punched a colleague before, but I'm about to make an exception as well."

Sebastian raised his hands in mock surrender. "Take it easy, sunshine. I was just joking around."

Kiernan swung his arm in Sebastian's direction, prompting him to lurch back from the counter with a high-pitched yelp.

Instead of landing a punch, Kiernan patted him on the shoulder. "You're awfully jumpy today. Might want to cut back on your morning caffeine fix."

With a wink, Kiernan headed off for a quick chat with Dr. Fleming.

Jan Reddy was lying down on the treatment table when Kiernan entered the room. Her face was turned away as she stared at the far wall, but upon hearing the door swing open, she immediately looked over.

"Hello, Jan, I'm Mr. O'Rourke," Kiernan said as he walked up to her and shook her hand. "I'm the chief of surgery here at West Mercy." He pulled up a chair and seated himself close to the head of the table. "My staff have been keeping me up to date on your case, but I wanted to meet and talk to you personally, if that's okay."

Her tense face softened into a smile. "Yes, of course."

"I know these past few days since the spina bifida diagnosis haven't been easy."

She shook her head. "They haven't. You read about this sort of thing happening to other women, and you never think it's going to happen to you. Especially since my other two pregnancies were perfectly healthy."

"Unfortunately, that's how it is sometimes with birth defects. There's no rhyme or reason to it. I reviewed your case history, and you have none of the risk factors."

"That's what Dr. Fleming said. She's so nice… But things like diabetes, and I think she said folate deficiency was another factor—they don't apply to me."

Kiernan pressed his lips together and nodded. At times like this, when there was nothing he could do in the moment to instantly fix something, he could only offer a genuine gesture of understanding.

"So, I know Dr. Fleming has talked to you about fetal surgery to repair the spinal opening…"

"She has. And I know the surgery can't be done here."

"Believe me when I say I wish that weren't the case. We're working hard to get to a point where we can offer fetal surgeries for spina bifida and other congenital anomalies. In the meantime, we're hoping we can find a spot for you at another hospital that can perform this procedure. I spoke to Dr. Fleming a little while ago, and she said that even if we can, you have some concerns about whether to move forward with the surgery."

"I do. And I know this probably won't make any sense, but when I found out that I was a candidate for fetal surgery, I wished for a second that I wasn't. Because that way I wouldn't have to make a decision that could possibly lead to the death of my baby." She paused and swallowed hard. "Or me. And I want you to know that I would do anything to save my baby's life—even if it meant losing mine. But I have two other children who need me. And a husband, too." She rolled her eyes, topped off with a half-smile. "You know how most men are just big babies themselves."

Kiernan laughed quietly. "So I've heard."

He truly felt for Jan. She was facing a dilemma that he wouldn't wish on anyone. It was true that not all mothers-to-be facing her predicament fulfilled the criteria needed to move forward with the surgery. From the mother's past medical history to a current BMI, and even the presence of a support person, there were a number of boxes that needed to be checked off before the green light could be given for the procedure. Additionally, the anomaly had to be discovered early enough for the surgery to be performed—in the twenty-second to twenty-fifth week of pregnancy. In Jan's case, it had been discovered during her second trimester scan at twenty-one weeks. Which meant the clock was ticking… and the pressure was on.

As a surgeon, Kiernan didn't believe in sugarcoating the risks to a patient. In his mind, it was ultimately a disservice to them. Instead, he believed they should have all the facts they needed to make an informed decision, and he would always fully support them in whatever they chose to do.

"Jan, I know this is not an easy decision. I'm sure Dr. Fleming went over this with you, but there's always the option of post-delivery surgery. This would typically be within the first twenty-four to forty-eight hours after birth. It's less risky but, since spina bifida is a progressive condition, it won't halt progression within the womb like fetal surgery can do, so your baby will most likely experience more complications down the road. That being said, I've seen it lessen considerably the severity of spina bifida in the handful of patients that we've treated here."

"And you can perform this surgery here?"

"Yes."

"But it won't fix the defect to the same degree that fetal surgery can?"

"Unfortunately, no."

Jan stared up at the ceiling and sighed. "I wish I could talk to someone who's actually performed fetal surgery for spina bifida and can personally share with me the good and bad of how it turned out." She gasped, then sat up on her elbows. "I'm sorry, Mr. O'Rourke! I didn't mean to imply that talking to you isn't helpful, because it is…"

Kiernan smiled. "No need to apologize. I totally understand where you're coming from. I'm still hopeful that we'll be able to line you up with a surgeon at another hospital, and once we do, I'm sure they'll be more than happy to answer any of your questions."

She squeezed her lips together as though doing her best to smile through her anxious thoughts. "Thank you for coming by."

"Of course." Kiernan stood up. "And I know you're in good hands with Dr. Fleming and the rest of her team, but I'm here if you need anything."

This time her smile was full width. "I appreciate that."

As Kiernan started down the hospital corridor, he tried to organize the tidal wave of thoughts that were cresting all at once in his mind. Hearing Jan speak firsthand about the treatment options for her baby's condition only strengthened his resolve to ensure West Mercy's new neonatal wing would one day be fully equipped to offer cutting-edge fetal surgery—and more.

But that wasn't going to help Jan now. His temples throbbed with the realization that, no matter how lofty his ambitions to go all in and give one hundred and ten percent on behalf of his patients, there were still obstacles that he had no control over. All he could do was plow ahead, knowing that progress was inevitable, but often on its own timetable.

And then another thought hit him like a bolt of lightning. He paused and rifled through the pocket of his lab coat, extracting his phone and instantly initiating a search. Tapping on a search results link, his eyes widened…and then widened some more.

"Thank you, Sebastian," he said under his breath. "You're a pain in the ass, but sometimes a *helpful* pain in the ass."

Claire tossed some breadcrumbs into the water and laughed as a small flock of ducks pounced on the treats, slurping them up within seconds. She threw out another handful, then announced, "That's all I got, guys!"

Yesterday, she had followed the path from her cottage down over a slight hill, through thickened brush and finally an opening that revealed the shallow, rocky shoreline of the bay. She had been instantly captivated by the colorful waterfowl, chirping birds and myriad wildflowers, and today was no different.

Despite her vow a few days ago to get out and mingle with other people, she was finding the quiet serenity of nature to be a much greater draw. Spotting a large boulder to sit on, she pulled up her knees and rested her forearms and chin on top of them. There was no doubt in her mind that this peaceful solitude would be a better facilitator than loud tourist spots for the monumental career decision that she needed to make. And yet she felt no closer to a resolution than when she had first arrived in the country.

Closing her eyes, she replayed all that had already transpired in less than a week. An emergency breech delivery. An unexpected but powerful attraction to a fellow doctor. No wonder she was no further along in sorting out a difficult professional dilemma.

Reopening her eyes and staring out at the gently shimmering waters, her thoughts were pulled like a magnet back to her encounter with Kiernan at the pub. Since the end of her marriage, and the loss of Ariana, she had not felt even the slightest spark of interest toward another man. Not those who had approached her during occasional social outings with friends, a drink in one hand and a "How *you* doing?" tumbling out of their mouths, nor the male colleagues who had been circling the waters upon news of her divorce.

Her therapist and her friends had more than once suggested that maybe she was protecting her heart after Mark's betrayal and Ariana's death. But if that were true, it was on an unconscious level, rather than a deliberate decision to squash any attraction. She simply hadn't *felt* anything, either physically or emotionally, toward another man. And, given that she hadn't been in the right headspace to open her heart up to someone else, it was probably just as well.

And yet, with seemingly no effort on his part, Kiernan had drawn her in and reawakened a yearning in her that she had come to believe was gone for good. Perhaps it was the easy rapport they shared. The kind brown eyes and disarming smile. The sexily tousled hair—oh, heck, the sexy *everything*. She smiled at the deliciousness of her thoughts— until reminding herself that although daydreaming about Kiernan was an enjoyable pastime, it was also a distraction that she couldn't afford right now. Not when her career hung in the balance, and her time would be best spent engaging in some serious soul-searching.

With that in mind, Claire forced herself to re-direct her thoughts. But a sudden, familiar voice stopped them dead in their tracks.

"Claire!"

Swinging her head around, Claire watched, mouth slightly agape, as Kiernan spread aside the end of a thicket patch with both hands and emerged out into the open.

What in the...?

She stood up from the boulder, both happy to see

him and wishing she could feel otherwise. "How in the world did you know where to find me?"

Kiernan grinned, the sun catching golden flecks in his brown eyes. "Well, I knocked on every pink cottage door, and only strangers answered. Then I came to your cottage, and no one was home. But I saw fresh footprints that looked to be your size on the path behind the cottage and decided to follow them."

"For real," she insisted, with a *Yeah, right* expression etched across her face.

"Okay, the red Mini parked outside gave it away."

Claire tapped her head with her hand as if to say, *Of course.*

"I know this is a surprise…" Kiernan said, taking a few more steps to close the gap between them.

"You could say that."

Kiernan stared into her eyes. "I have a favor to ask you. Actually, if you could magnify the word 'favor' by about ten thousand, then that's what I'm about to ask."

"Okay, now you're starting to scare me," Claire said, only half kidding.

"I don't mean to scare you," Kiernan said, as he briefly touched her forearm.

Perhaps the gesture was meant to calm her, but the electricity that shot through her had the opposite effect. Coupled with the intense physical attraction she felt for the hunky surgeon just inches away from her, the surge caught her off guard. But as she regained her breath and looked into his eyes, she allowed herself to settle into the feeling his touch provoked. And it felt good.

"I met with a patient today whose unborn baby was recently diagnosed with spina bifida."

Kiernan's words quickly put a damper on the opening she had allowed herself. She wasn't sure if it was her chest or her stomach that tightened first, but either way a sense of dread was building.

"She's been ruled as a candidate for fetal surgery, and we're trying to set her up with a hospital that offers the procedure. But she's worried about the outcome if she goes through with it. She has two young children, and she doesn't want to leave them without a mother if something goes wrong."

"There's always a risk," Claire conceded, "but the odds would still be in her favor."

"I think knowing that would help her make the right decision for her baby and her family."

"You mean no doctors at West Mercy have explained the risks and benefits of the surgery to her?"

"They have. But I really think it would help if she heard it from someone who's actually performed the procedure."

Claire felt her heart quicken—no small feat given that her chest was now tighter than a drum. "Wait—do you mean *me*?"

Kiernan nodded, his eyes eager with anticipation.

"What makes you think I've even performed this surgery?"

"It came up in a Google search."

"You *Googled* me?" Claire asked, her voice rising.

"It's not as bad as it sounds," Kiernan replied, his face tight as though he were talking on eggshells, never mind walking on them.

"After meeting with the patient this morning—her name is Jan—I got to wondering if maybe you'd done this sort of surgery yourself. It was just a hunch. In fact, I wasn't expecting anything to turn up in my search when I entered your name, but quite a bit did." He paused, his face softening as he added, "It's not my fault you're an exceptionally talented doctor."

Claire *almost* smiled.

"You've performed close to a dozen successful spina bifida fetal surgeries. I mean, I can't imagine anyone more qualified to talk to Jan about what to expect if she moves forward with the surgery." He paused, the silence between them peppered with the sound of birdsong and water gently lapping up against rocks. "I know you're here on vacation, and I shouldn't even be asking you. But if you're up for this, it would just be an hour at most of your time. A consultation, that's all."

Claire stared down at the ground as she ran through the scenario in her head.

A woman has discovered she's carrying a baby with a condition that could significantly compromise the quality of his or her life. She's devastated. She's scared. She wants to do the right thing for her unborn baby and the two children she already

*has. How can I not do what I can to help her make
that decision?*

Claire knew very well that she couldn't answer this question without first placing it within a
greater context. After all, if there were two things
that were *not* on her Ireland travel itinerary, they
were entering a hospital and meeting with a patient.
Especially when her whole reason for being here
was to figure out whether she could resume that
life. But there was a flipside to every coin, and an
argument could just as easily be made that the only
way to determine this would be to walk the walk.
Which in this case meant meeting Jan and talking
through the treatment options that were best for
her and her unborn baby.

Trial by fire. Or, better yet, trial by *controlled*
fire.

Claire looked back up at Kiernan, silently catching her breath as his handsome face greeted her
with a smile. There was something in that moment between them that told her she could do this.
Something about *him* that made her feel safe and
infused with inner strength.

"Okay," she said, a smile slowly emerging. "I'll
do it."

"Thank you," Kiernan said breathlessly. "Thank
you so much."

"No need to thank me."

"Would tomorrow work for you?" he asked. "Say
at around eleven a.m.?"

"Yes, I can do that."

"Great! I'll pick you up at—"

"I'll drive to the hospital myself," Claire interjected, softening her tone when she noticed how Kiernan flinched at her unintended harshness.

It was difficult enough pushing past her fears and agreeing to the consultation. No need to add to the stomach butterflies she'd be feeling tomorrow by sitting oh-so-close to Kiernan on the drive in.

"After all, I've got this cute little Mini, so I might as well put it to use."

Kiernan chuckled. "Yes, good idea."

Ten silent seconds passed by as slow as molasses. Claire smiled and widened her eyes—her go-to expression when she was feeling uneasy or awkward. There was a nonverbal exchange of...*something*...between them, and it pulled at every fiber of her being in a way that she hadn't felt in a very long time.

"So I'll see you and Jan tomorrow at eleven?" she asked, feeling the need to fill in the silence.

Kiernan smiled and nodded—then jolted slightly as though suddenly remembering something. He pulled his phone from a side pocket in his scrub pants. "Should we exchange phone numbers? Just in case there's an emergency or I need to adjust the time?"

Claire hesitated momentarily. It was a reasonable request, but also one more swing of the sledgehammer into the barrier she had built around herself. But maybe she should let go of a brick or two. For Kiernan, she could do that.

"My phone is in the cottage, but call my number and I'll have yours as well." She quickly recited the numbers, and he punched them into his phone.

"Great. Well, I've got two surgeries scheduled this afternoon, so I'd better be heading back to the hospital." He started to leave, then stopped. "Oh, and don't forget. We drive on the left side of the road here."

Claire grinned. "Thanks for the reminder."

Trudging through the dense thicket that lined the midsection of the path on the way back to his car, Kiernan felt elated. Not even the thorns that were catching on his shirt or the burrs sticking to his hair were enough to deter his ear-to-ear smile. He had successfully convinced Claire to meet with Jan and fully trusted that she would help Jan better understand the risks and benefits of spina bifida fetal surgery so that she could make the best possible decision for her and her family.

But his smile soon wavered as he replayed the look in Claire's eyes as he had awaited her answer. Granted, he hadn't expected her to jump for joy at the prospect of taking time out of her vacation to consult on a patient. Or…maybe he kind of had. She was a dedicated doctor and a confident, highly skilled surgeon, and this was an opportunity to weigh in on a potential surgical outcome that could significantly better the lives of a mother and her unborn child. Plus, shouldn't she be even mildly curious to see how West Mercy was positioning itself to eventually offer innovative neonatal surgeries? So why the unmistakable hesitancy on her part?

His hand resting on the door handle of his SUV, Kiernan stood immobile as he pondered the question further. Finally, he shook his head and opened the door. Perhaps he was overthinking things. His question had caught Claire by surprise, and understandably so. Tomorrow it would all work out. Jan would get the consultation she had hoped for. And he would once again have the chance to bask in Claire's presence. And, oh, what a presence it was. Beauty, intelligence, empathy and compassion—all wrapped into one somewhat mysterious but altogether magnetic package.

His thoughts were steamrollering through his head—until an obvious buzzkill slammed on the brakes. In less than a month Claire would be returning to her life in the States. Which meant time was of the essence if he was going to act on his undeniable attraction to her. Perhaps Sebastian was right—painful as that was to admit. He should savor the present moment—nothing more, nothing less. And the good thing about the present moment? It was already here.

CHAPTER FIVE

CLAIRE FELT HER tight grip on the steering wheel relax as late-morning sunshine filtered in through the Mini's windshield and side windows. The fact that she had butterflies in her stomach was more than apropos, given that springtime was on the verge of full bloom in the early-May countryside.

The serene landscape of lush fields and colorful wildflowers helped calm her nerves, but didn't erase them altogether. Not that anything could totally put her at ease. After all, she was on her way to West Mercy Hospital, where she would be meeting with a worried mother to help her make a momentous decision about her unborn baby.

You can do this, Claire told herself, slowly drawing in a breath of air and holding it for several moments as she inwardly repeated the mantra. *It's a one-time consultation, that's all.*

She needed to remind herself of this as well, given that it was a far cry from her normal interaction with patients. She was accustomed to getting to know them and their families well—especially those who were dealing with difficult medical situations.

The importance of maintaining an emotional detachment had been instilled in her since day one of medical school. But even though she had been an overachiever in all of her classes, this was one area where she didn't mind falling short if it meant allowing herself to care about her patients. She celebrated their joys and grieved their losses. Only now did she realize how doing so had made it more difficult to put her own pain aside when she had resumed her physician duties after losing Ariana.

Driving into the West Mercy parking lot, she pulled into the nearest open space, turned off the engine, then closed her eyes and reminded herself that she needed to hide her vulnerability not just from Jan, but from Kiernan, too. Neither of them needed to know that she felt like a walking open wound. Or that just speaking the word "baby" was enough to grab at her gut with a pain that she actually felt on a physical level.

The good news was there could be a happy ending to all of this. As a onetime consultant on Jan's condition, she would be playing the most minor of roles in such a miracle, but it was still something.

Walking up to the main entrance a short time later, Claire suddenly stopped in her tracks and viewed the multi-building complex before her. Seen from the front, the hospital was much larger than she had expected, prompting inevitable reminders of Boston General. Her earlier resolve to push past potential triggers was facing its first severe test, and she had to quickly recover before all was lost.

Deep breaths. Deep breaths.

Pinching her palm with her nails, she temporarily dispersed the distressing thoughts and memories that were tumbling forth. A few more seconds, another deep breath, and she was fully back in the present.

Once inside the entrance, Claire realized she hadn't locked down the details of where exactly to meet Kiernan. But as she approached the main nurses' station, she recognized a familiar friendly face.

"Hello, Dr. Delaney," Lucy said with a warm smile as she walked out from behind the station counter. "Mr. O'Rourke has just finished with a patient and is on his way down." Glancing over her shoulder, she added, "Speak of the devil."

"Are you calling me the devil?" Kiernan asked with amusement as he seemingly materialized from out of the blue.

Or maybe Claire's slightly dizzy reaction upon seeing him once again just made it feel that way. It was a brief but altogether enjoyable distraction from her nerves.

Lucy flashed a side grin. "Of course not. You're nothing short of angelic, Mr. O'Rourke. And I know your patients would all agree."

"Good save." There was a twinkle in Kiernan's eyes that grew in intensity as he shifted his gaze to Claire. "How was the drive in?" he asked, his dark brown hair imperfectly…yet perfectly…tousled.

Claire's next breath caught in her throat. If ever there was an *I'm a brilliant surgeon too busy to brush my hair, but I'm still sexy as heck* vibe, then this had to be it. Not that Kiernan deliberately sent out those signals. Up to this point, everything in his demeanor had convinced Claire that he had no idea how attractive he was. Or, if he did, it fell so low on his list of important virtues that he simply couldn't care less.

She forced herself to exhale, then smiled. "It was fine. I have to say I really like that little Mini. I'm not sure how it would fare during a Boston winter, but I think I'm going to look into getting one when I'm back in the States."

Kiernan's smile momentarily faltered, as though the reminder of the temporary nature of her stay had triggered a somber moment. Or maybe she was just projecting her own suddenly mixed feelings on the subject.

Stepping off the elevator several minutes later, Kiernan turned to Claire. "Before you talk to Jan, I thought you might want to look over her case notes and test results."

Claire nodded. "Sure, that's a good idea."

"My office is just down this hall," he said.

Upon entering the smallish but neat and well-lit room, Claire's eyes were drawn to the barrage of diplomas and certificates, along with a handful of framed photos, that lined the wall behind his desk. "I can see you're quite the underachiever," she observed wryly.

Kiernan grinned slightly, but said nothing as

he rifled through a pile of folders on his expansive desk.

"Wait—is that Bono?" Claire asked incredulously as she homed in on a photo of Kiernan hugging shoulders with the Irish rocker.

Kiernan looked up from a thick folder that he had just extracted from the pile. "Ah, yes. That's from a hospital charity event last year. Quite an interesting chap—and very generous, too."

Claire eyed Kiernan curiously, amused by his rather nonchalant reply.

There was a knock on the partially open door, and she and Kiernan turned as a young male nurse in light green scrubs began to enter the room. Realizing that Kiernan wasn't alone, he stopped midstep.

"Sorry, I'll come back," he said, slowly retreating backwards.

"No, come on in," Kiernan said. "Did you hear back from UCLH?"

The man frowned, as though dreading his own reply. "I did. Mr. Ferguson dislocated his shoulder during a golf match over the weekend. He's out of commission for at least the next month."

"Damn," Kiernan muttered under his breath. "We're running out of options. And that one was looking like a sure thing." He sighed heavily, then turned back to the nurse. "What about Manchester General?"

"Still waiting to hear back."

"Okay, keep me posted."

"I will," the nurse said, before exiting the room.

Claire didn't want to pry about what was clearly distressing news for Kiernan, but she did wonder if it could possibly have something to do with Jan. She didn't have to guess for long.

"That was University College Hospital in London," Kiernan explained. "We were told a few days ago that they might be able to do Jan's surgery in two weeks. I haven't told her yet, because we were waiting for final confirmation, and it's a good thing I didn't. And I get grief for risking injury while playing rugby... Who knew putting a tiny white ball around in starched checked trousers was more dangerous than being face-deep in mud at the bottom of a rugby pileup?"

"Wild," Claire said quietly, viscerally feeling Kiernan's frustration. "But fetal surgery is more common now than, say, even ten years ago. Granted, not every hospital is equipped to perform some of the procedures, or has the right team in place, but it seems like there should be more options if you're expanding your search outside the country."

"There are. But one of the issues is red tape—something I'm sure you deal with back in America as well."

Claire rolled her eyes almost instinctively. "I have more experience with that than I'd like to admit. But I thought it would be a bit less so here, given the exchange between countries within Europe. Not that I fully understand how that might work."

"Unfortunately, red tape is red tape—especially when it comes to scheduling a complex surgery in another country at short notice." He grimaced, then gave a slight nod of the head as though trying to snap himself out of negative thoughts. "Here," he said, his voice softening as he handed the folder to Claire. "This should have all of Jan's records."

"Thanks," Claire replied, the hefty stack of papers landing in her hands like a solid brick. Or two. "You don't have digital records here at the hospital?"

"We do. But I like to have a hard copy of cases I'm working on as well." He paused, a half-smirk slowly emerging. "Call me old school."

Claire grinned. "Nothing wrong with that."

She leafed through the numerous documents in the folder, pausing at the ultrasound report. It confirmed what she'd expected with considerable apprehension: Jan's baby had the most severe form of spina bifida, myelomeningocele, in which part of the spine protruded from the back in a fluid-filled sac. It meant the surgery would be that much more difficult—and a positive outcome would be that much more life-enhancing. She then viewed the surgery criteria notes, a checklist of close to two dozen "must-haves" in order for the surgery to move forward. No history of placenta previa or hypertension…ability to adhere to a follow-up requirements…*check, check, check*….

It was only when she was three-quarters through the checklist that she realized she had been reviewing the notes without the stomach-churning anxiety she had tried to prepare for. Could it be because she was in a new hospital, and not at Boston General, which had triggers at every turn? It was a possible revelation that she'd need to ruminate on further. But right now she had to concentrate on Jan's prognosis.

Finishing her review, Claire looked up to find that Kiernan had been watching her intently, as though taking his next breath was contingent upon receiving her thumbs-up. She wasn't about to disappoint him.

"Jan's a textbook candidate for this surgery."

He pursed his lips together and nodded. "That's my team's assessment as well. But I wanted to hear it from the expert."

There was the slightest teasing edge to Kiernan's voice, but Claire didn't mind. She knew he respected her exceptional knowledge and experience on this matter—just as she respected his immense know-how in…well, no doubt in everything related to surgery and hospital leadership.

"Shall we go and talk to Jan?" Kiernan asked as he opened the door to the hallway and gestured for Claire to exit first.

Claire smiled, masking her inner turmoil. As she started down the hallway, with Kiernan by her side, there were only two thoughts in her mind:

Stay strong for Jan. And for her baby.

* * *

Kiernan ushered Claire into a tastefully decorated consultation room that more closely resembled a cozy parlor.

A petite woman in a white lab coat with a short black bob and ice-blue eyes immediately stood up from one of several thick-cushioned chairs and came over.

"I'm Dr. Fleming, senior doctor ob-gyn," she said, shaking Claire's hand. "Mr. O'Rourke has filled me in on everything, and I really appreciate you taking the time to talk to Jan about fetal surgery."

"Nice to meet you," Claire said.

As Dr. Fleming resumed her seat, Kiernan introduced Claire to Jan, who sat on the adjacent couch.

"Hi," she said, managing a weak smile. "Thank you for being here. Mr. O'Rourke said you're an expert at spina bifida fetal surgery."

Now seated between Dr. Fleming and Kiernan, Claire silently took note of the dark circles under Jan's eyes, the hollow cheeks and raspy voice. There was no doubt that the immense worry about her unborn baby's condition was taking its toll.

"I'm glad to be here," Claire replied. "I know Mr. O'Rourke and Dr. Fleming have talked to you about the benefits of fetal surgery for your baby, and I'm sure you have lots of questions."

"I do. But the two main ones are, will it work? And is there a possibility I won't survive the surgery?" Jan's voice cracked as she added, "I'm not asking about survival for myself. I'm asking for the sake of my other two children."

Claire gripped the armrest of her chair as the air seemed to suddenly evaporate from the room. She wanted so badly to be fully present for Jan, to calm her fears and help her make the right choice for *all* her children. But first she needed to push past her own lingering trauma.

From the corner of her eye, she could see Kiernan's forehead crease as he glanced down at her white-knuckled grasp of the chair-arm. She had to rein in her emotions, or the situation would quickly spiral downwards.

Focus, Claire, focus...

Pulling herself back to the present, Claire explained to Jan that the rigorous screening process would help ensure the surgery's safety and success. And with each additional question Jan posed, Claire dug deep within herself to stay in the moment. By the time Jan got around to asking whether her previous spina bifida surgeries had been successful nearly twenty minutes had passed, and Claire's anxiety was almost fully in check.

"Here," Claire said after scrolling briefly through her phone and pulling up a picture. She quickly showed the image to Kiernan and Dr. Fleming before walking over to Jan. "This is Samantha. Her mom sent me this picture a few months ago, when Samantha turned five. She was one of my first fetal surgery patients, and she's doing great. Her mom said she started school last fall, and is keeping right up with the other kids."

Jan leaned in further to get a closer look at the young girl with blonde pigtails, freckles and an ear-to-ear smile. "And if she hadn't had the surgery it might have been a different outcome—right?"

Claire reluctantly nodded. Her whole purpose for coming here today was to help steer Jan in the direction that she truly felt was best for her and her unborn child. But if no hospital was available to do the surgery in time, then what was the point? She'd be doing little more than confirming to Jan that her best option was unobtainable. Without the surgery, Jan's unborn baby faced a host of potential health issues, including incontinence, paralysis and cognitive impairment.

Claire turned to Kiernan, meeting his eyes and feeling that he somehow understood her dilemma. He quickly stepped in and reassured Jan that they were doing everything they could to schedule the surgery at an appropriate facility. But would it happen in time? Claire wanted to stay optimistic, but doubt was setting in. She was used to preparing herself for the possibility that a treatment option might fall short of the desired outcome, especially for a high-risk pregnancy. But to not even have the chance to get a life-enhancing surgery off the ground?

That possibility brought with it a new sense of helplessness that she wasn't accustomed to.

* * *

"That seemed to go well," Kiernan said later, as he and Claire walked down the hospital corridor after the consultation had ended.

Claire nodded, but couldn't quite muster up a smile.

Kiernan eyed her sideways as they turned onto another corridor. "You're not saying much."

"Sorry. I think it went well, too. But unfortunately, I feel like maybe all I did was get her hopes up for a surgery that she might not be able to get in time."

Kiernan sighed. "I know. I was kind of fighting that thought as well. She did say she'd be willing to travel further than she initially indicated, so I'm going to tell my team to expand their search outside of Ireland and the UK Or I should say outside of the UK It's already been confirmed nothing can be scheduled in time at the few facilities equipped for this surgery in Ireland."

"But it's not just the surgery—there's all the follow-up, too. And it could mean being away from her children for quite some time."

"I thought of that as well. But Dr. Fleming is getting her team up to speed on post-surgery care for Jan. She thinks it can be handled here, especially with the neonatal unit fully operational."

"I thought you said it wasn't open yet?"

"Not officially. But construction is completed, and the operating theaters and patient wards are equipped and ready to go." He turned to Claire as they continued their walk. "You know how hospital boards are. They want the opening to be big on publicity and fanfare."

"Is that what you want?"

"Personally, I couldn't care less about all that stuff." As they came to a large sliding glass door at the end of the corridor, Kiernan slowed to a halt, with Claire following his lead. "I just want to start offering cutting-edge neonatal care here, so we don't have to scramble to find other options for patients like Jan. But I'm also pragmatic enough to realize that we need to get the word out on as large a scale as possible to make this new undertaking a success. We can't help women with high-risk pregnancies if they're not being sent here for treatment. And that will only happen when we start forging a reputation for top-tier neonatal care."

"Good point."

Claire wondered if the intense effort behind her smile was obvious to Kiernan. She hoped it wasn't. In another time and place she'd be excited to talk about advanced treatment options for high-risk pregnancies. Heck, it was the type of conversation that she herself once typically initiated with colleagues. But that had been before the subject matter had become inextricably tied to personal loss and pain.

Kiernan turned and swiped his badge along the reader. The glass doors swiftly opened, and he gestured to Claire to enter first.

She wrinkled her nose slightly as they started

down the corridor. "It almost has that new car smell in here."

Kiernan eyed her curiously from the side. "Funny you picked up on that. It's because everything *is* new in here. This is the neonatal wing I've been talking your ear off about."

Claire's breath caught in her throat, her rapid walk quickly decelerating.

Kiernan slowed down with her, his face perplexed. "Are you okay?"

Claire inwardly scrambled to salvage the situation. With every fiber of her being she wanted to avoid being pulled further back into the world of pregnancies and babies. Yes, she was at West Mercy today by choice. But she had never intended for her visit to extend beyond her consultation with Jan.

Still…could she reframe this moment? See it as an opportunity to witness a hospital making major progress for women's health and that of their newborn babies? Confirm to Kiernan that he was doing a commendable thing by driving this progress? He deserved no less. And perhaps at the same time she could begin to see glimpses of the joy and satisfaction she had once derived from playing an integral role in the health and wellness of mothers and their babies.

She looked up at him. His eyes were still searching hers. "I'm okay," she finally replied, conjuring up a smile as she gestured to the corridor before them. "Lead the way."

Kiernan appeared more than happy to oblige. Weaving through the main areas of the wing with Claire at his side, he paused at intervals to get her input on a particular process or piece of medical apparatus, as though wanting to ensure no stone had been left unturned in his quest for the most advanced neonatal center possible.

Entering the neonatal intensive care unit, Claire braced herself for an onslaught of emotion. A startled technician turned from the incubator that he had been testing with a biomedical analyzer. As Kiernan engaged him in a friendly conversation Claire held her breath, wondering if an anxiety episode was about to burst forth. But instead, the tightness in her chest dissipated, and she found herself peering more closely at the state-of-the-art equipment.

Could it be because the memories of her last moments with Ariana were confined to a birthing room and had never progressed to the NICU? Possibly. She only knew that she felt a sense of relief to have made it this far without any significant emotional fallout.

"And that concludes your personalized tour of the new West Mercy neonatal wing," Kiernan said twenty minutes later as they circled back to their starting point. "I hope you've enjoyed this sneak peek of our soon-to-open cutting-edge unit, and please come back again soon."

Her initial raw nerves had now dialed down several notches, and Claire couldn't help but snicker at Kiernan's pitch-perfect flight attendant voice.

"Well done," she conceded. "I can see why you're proud of this unit. Everything is state of the art, and once your team is certified in some of the specialized neonatal and fetal surgery techniques, I can't imagine West Mercy won't make a name for itself in neonatal medicine."

"I'm glad you think so," Kiernan said, looking pleased. "Yours is a highly coveted opinion."

The line was delivered with both sincerity and a touch of humor, and Claire laughed in return.

A door opened behind Kiernan and an electrician emerged, with a flashlight in one hand and a workbag in the other. He pulled the *Do Not Enter* sign off the door, then addressed Kiernan.

"All set, sir. There was some loose wiring in one of the walls, but I reconnected it and everything's good to go."

"Great," Kiernan said, turning to Claire. "The birthing suites are down this way. I didn't think I'd be able to show you, since there's been some electrical issues and we closed off the area out of an abundance of caution, but it looks like we've got the green light."

Before Claire could come up with an excuse to pass on this final and most potentially triggering leg of the tour, Kiernan swung open the door.

"You first."

Moments later they were standing inside a spacious yet cozy birthing suite. Soothing rays of natural light filtered in through floor-to-ceiling windows, dancing off the earth-toned walls and casting an iridescent glow over vast paintings of pastoral landscapes.

The scene was eerily familiar, and as Claire's eyes darted around the room a heavy sadness descended upon her.

Five and a half months into her pregnancy, she and Mark had stood in a nearly identical room during a birthing suite tour at Boston General, admiring the suite's calming color scheme and expansive windows.

Or, at least, *she* had viewed the surroundings with awe. Mark, on the other hand, had seemed distant and distracted. She recalled the unease she had felt at his I-want-to-be-anywhere-but-here vibe, chalking it up at the time to the jitters of impending fatherhood.

But even then, something in the pit of her stomach told her there was more at play. Unable to fathom that her suspicions could possibly be true, she had squelched her snowballing doubts.

When they had solidified into reality less than a month later with his abrupt departure, the snowballs had turned into an avalanche of disbelief.

Needing something to grab on to, Claire searched for the nearest solid object. *Kiernan.* No, she was not going to grasp his arm, regardless of how muscular and strong it appeared to be. He might be wearing a lab coat now, but a form-fitting rugby shirt hid no secrets, and she wasn't about to forget *that* earlier image anytime soon.

Really? You're thinking about Kiernan's hunk of a build now?

Mind racing, Claire tried to reason with herself, but crazy thoughts had a way of quickly multiplying. Sweat beads broke out on her forehead. She had almost made it through the tour unscathed. *Almost.* If only the electrician's exit had been delayed a few more minutes. Then she and Kiernan would have moved on from the area and....

"Claire?" Kiernan said, alarm in his voice.

She peered up at him, wondering if she looked like a deer in the headlights, ready to bolt. That was certainly how she felt.

"You're awfully pale. Sit down," he said, nodding to a plump-pillowed chair against the wall. "Let me get you some water."

"I think I… I just need some air."

Making a beeline for the door, Claire was only half aware that Kiernan was right on her heels. But when he jumped in front of her out in the hallway, she could no longer pretend she was unraveling sight unseen. Kiernan had a front row seat to her meltdown, and her humiliation was only equaled by her desire to be instantly transported off the hospital grounds.

Wrapping his arm around her shoulder, Kiernan began to steer her diagonally toward a door on the other side of the corridor. With her fight-or-flight response switched on—emphasis on flight—Claire wanted to run for the nearest exit. But Kiernan's strong, protective grip was like a weighted blanket cocooned around her, and her rapid shallow breathing began to slow down a notch.

Once inside the empty exam room, Kiernan gently helped Claire onto a chair, then pulled another chair up beside her. He placed her hand over the palm side of his wrist, then draped his other hand on top of it.

"Just breathe and feel my pulse, and let yours sync to it."

Thump...thump...thump...

Claire closed her eyes and allowed Kiernan's slow, steady heartbeat to seep deeply into her very being. She felt her shoulders drop, and for the first time became aware that her feet were touching the ground. It was as if his strong but calm heartbeat was telling her own rapid-fire pulse: *Just follow me and everything will be okay.*

When she finally opened her eyes and looked up at Kiernan, she couldn't be sure how much time had passed. She only knew that his kind brown eyes were gazing deeply into own.

"I think we need to trade hearts," she quipped, her weakened voice cracking slightly.

The earlier adrenaline coursing through her body had been the equivalent of running a marathon, but at least she had crossed the finish line—and all thanks to the handsome surgeon just inches away from her.

"There's nothing wrong with your heart at all,"

Kiernan replied, with such decisiveness that she couldn't help but feel he wasn't just referring to its physical aspects.

Mr. O'Rourke, please report to Room 247 for a consultation.

Claire looked up at the intercom box above the doorway, then back at Kiernan.

He shook his head. "It can wait. You're my patient now."

A smile slowly emerged, and he squeezed her hand just tightly enough for her heart to skip a beat. He sure had a way of making her heart do unexpected things.

"I'm feeling much better," she finally managed to say. "Thank you."

"No need to thank me."

"I should let you get back to work."

"I'm not leaving until I'm certain you're okay." He cocked his head slightly to one side, as if wondering whether to say more. "Is there anything you want to talk about? My colleagues like to call me a grump behind my back—and sometimes to my face, for that matter—but truth be told, I'm a really good listener."

Claire smirked. "I'm sure you are. But I'm okay—really. I should have mentioned that I can be sensitive to a lot of environmental things. I probably just had a reaction to the new paint or the carpets in the suite."

She could tell by Kiernan's narrowed eyes that

he wasn't buying her excuse for a second. But that didn't stop her from doubling down.

"Besides, you know how we doctors make the worst patients. Once I'm outside and get some fresh air, I'll be good as new."

"Well, let me at least walk you out to your car."

"That's not necessary—"

"I insist," Kiernan interjected, his sternness offset by the twinkle in his eye. "Besides, I'm going to be checking your stride. Any wobbliness and you'll be confined to quarters."

"Confined to quarters?" Claire repeated with a touch of amusement in her voice. "Is this a hospital or a military institution?"

Kiernan let out a mock sigh. "Sometimes it feels like a little of both."

The rejuvenating midday sun felt good on Claire's face as she walked through the parking lot to her car, with Kiernan close by her side.

"Are you sure you're okay?" he asked as she seated herself in the Mini and rolled down the window.

She smiled. "I'm sure."

"Thank you again for talking to Jan."

"Happy to do so."

After an exchange of goodbyes, Claire watched as Kiernan strode confidently across the parking lot, waiting for him to disappear from view before leaning her head back against the seat and taking a deep breath. She closed her eyes, wishing more than anything that his hand could still be clasping her own as her heartbeat synched with his. How he had turned the feeling of a pulse—normally just a routine diagnostic tool—into something so...*intimate* was something she'd be pondering for days to come.

But it was more than that. He had stayed with her, offering to talk about what had triggered her reaction and refusing to leave her side until he was convinced she was okay. And the kicker to all of this? Not once had he made her feel like he was doing so out of medical obligation.

Compare that to Mark, who hadn't even made the effort to be present during the loss of their daughter....

Claire shook her head. *Don't go there.* A few more deep breaths. *Focus on the positive.*

It was easy enough to do. She just had to think of Kiernan, and the way she was starting to feel whenever he was near.

Up in the third-floor cafeteria, which offered the most expansive view of the parking lot below, Kiernan stared out of the floor-to-ceiling window, his eyes glued to Claire's red Mini. Though ten minutes had passed, it had yet to leave its parking spot, and he decided to give it one more minute before heading back outside to check on her.

Another twenty seconds and the Mini backed out and headed toward the exit. Kiernan stared at the empty spot for several moments, trying to wrap his head around what had just transpired. He had previously toyed with the possibility that there was more to Claire's story than her *I'm just taking a month-long vacation* declaration. But now his suspicions were deepening.

"Mr. O'Rourke to Theater Three, STAT."

The intercom announcement pulled him back to the present. With a possible emergency unfolding, he had to put those thoughts on hold. Although something told him they'd return soon enough…

CHAPTER SIX

KIERNAN KNOCKED BRIEFLY on the hospital room door, then entered while scanning patient notes on his tablet. Yesterday, his concerned speculation over a possible trauma in Claire's past had been cut short when he'd been summoned to the operating theater for a woman—Darla—who had just been admitted with a burst appendix. Always a perilous situation, the risk had been magnified tenfold because Darla was six months pregnant.

Fortunately, Darla's surgery had gone well, and she was now resting comfortably with her husband at her bedside, along with their two adolescent daughters.

"I just wanted to check in to see how you're doing," Kiernan said now, as Darla and her husband smiled appreciatively.

A few more minutes of friendly small talk and then Kiernan wished Darla a speedy recovery back home, knowing she'd be discharged later in the afternoon.

Exiting the room, he glanced back at the family once more, wincing slightly as he tried to suppress the wave of poignancy that descended over him. There was something eerily familiar about the scene, and he didn't have to dig deep within his memories to make the connection.

Twenty years ago, the heavily pregnant woman with a perforated appendix had been none other than his mother. He recalled his aunt bringing him and his younger sister Colleen to visit her during an extended hospital stay due to complications. And his father? He'd been nowhere to be found. Actually…that wasn't true. He'd been in the same hospital as Kiernan's mother, but too tied up with his patients to check in on the most important patient… the most important *person*…of all.

It was probably just as well, Kiernan thought now, eyes narrowing and jaw clenching as he quickened his pace down the corridor. It wasn't like his father had been known for his bedside manner— though for the patients whose lives he had saved, forgoing the warm fuzzies was probably considered a small price to pay.

Still, Kiernan had never forgotten the excuses his mother had made for his father's cruel absence when she'd needed him most. "Your father's busy saving other lives," she had said at the time, struggling to form a smile with parched lips nearly as pale as her anemic skin.

And she had been right. His father *had* been saving other lives. Which would have been all fine and dandy if he'd had no family of his own that needed him, too.

Perhaps that explained Kiernan's actions when his mother had been hospitalized at West Mercy with double pneumonia, just over a year ago. Though she hadn't been a surgical patient, he had popped into her room at every opportunity, plumping up her pillows, double-checking her meds and fussing over her like only a loving son-slash-doctor could.

"I'll say one thing," his mum had said during one such occasion, when his doting had been in full overdrive. "Maybe it's because I'm your mother, but you most definitely have much more of a bedside manner than your father ever did." She had paused, in part to take more air into her healing lungs but also to flash a rueful smile. "Thank goodness for that."

So at least he'd got that part right—and without any real effort, given that he truly cared about his patients. They were actual people, with hopes and dreams and loved ones, not merely a list of symptoms and diagnoses. But sidestepping his father's other major flaw... That required more deliberation on his part.

Throw himself into his career as a surgeon dedicated to saving lives? *Check.* Avoid serious personal relationships that would make that first goal impossible? *Check.* Because the two had to go together—right? Even his mother had seemed to think so. She'd never actually *said* this to him... rather it was more about what she hadn't said.

Once, several years ago, she had asked him when he was planning to settle down and start a family.

"You mean so I can be an absentee husband and father like Dad?" he had replied pointedly.

She had silently looked back at him, understanding and regret in her eyes. And she'd never asked again.

Back in his office, Kiernan stared at the wall as thoughts of Claire incessantly flooded his mind. Ever since they had parted ways yesterday, he had not been able to stop thinking about her. He had texted her last night, to see how she was feeling, and had been at least mildly relieved when she had replied that she was fine. But he wasn't fully convinced.

He closed his eyes, reliving each second that had ticked by when she had tuned in to his pulse, her hand delicately placed on his wrist and her beautiful face just inches away from him. Only now did he realize how lucky he had been that his heart rate hadn't surged with her touch. He had felt it quicken, and only through sheer willpower had he slowed it down so that she, too, would begin to relax.

With a loud sigh, Kiernan swung his chair around to stare at the other equally bland wall. What he wouldn't give to see her again. As in *now*.

Extracting his phone from his white coat, he stared at the screen, then quickly typed out a text before he could talk himself out of it.

There's a great little garden tea shop that serves lunch halfway between the hospital and your cottage. Fancy taking out the Mini to meet me there at noon?

Kiernan wasn't aware that he was holding his breath while waiting for the beep of a text reply from Claire. It was only when his screen lit up with the word Sure that he sputtered and realized he was probably turning blue.

Wonderful. I'll text you the address shortly.

Leaning back in his chair, Kiernan replenished his oxygen supply with some deep breaths, then shook his head slightly, perplexed by his own actions. Lunch—if he even paused long enough to have it—was typically a couple of power bars eaten while on the move from one patient or operating theater to the next. And now he was taking a chunk of time out of his busy schedule to meet Claire? And not just at any restaurant, mind you. By choosing a quaint little tea shop nestled within carefully manicured gardens of tulips, daffodils and roses, he was fully setting the scene for... Well, it couldn't be romance...could it?

"That's crazy talk," he muttered aloud to his own thoughts.

But as he launched himself out of the chair he felt nearly giddy at the thought of soon seeing Claire. It was a state of mind that was new to him. But what the heck.

I might as well go with it.

* * *

Kiernan waved to Claire as she approached the small white wrought-iron table on the outside patio of the Gilded Petal Tea Shop. He stood up and pulled out her chair, his nerve-endings on fire as her shiny chestnut hair fluttered against his forearm while he helped push her chair back in.

"You dressed for the occasion," he said, admiring the gauzy flowered dress that clung to her taut curves. Or maybe it was the curves themselves that he was admiring. He cleared his throat at the distinction.

Claire smirked as she nodded toward him. "And I see you didn't."

He glanced down at his green scrubs—an unfashionable necessity given he was squeezing in lunch between surgeries. "You never know when a wilted tulip is going to need medical intervention."

Claire's lilting laughter filtered through him like a soul-soothing elixir. It was a relief to find that the sparkle had returned to her eyes and the peachy glow to her cheeks. Perhaps he had prematurely jumped to conclusions about her puzzling reaction in the birthing suite.

"It's good to see you," he said. "Even though you said you felt okay when you left yesterday, you still had me worried."

Claire twisted her mouth to one side. "Like I said…doctors make the worst patients."

He grinned. "Well, I can't say I disagree with that."

A waitress came by and poured two cups of tea, placing a pot on the table and handing small, folded menus to each of them.

"I should have known this was one of those finger sandwich kinds of places," Kiernan said with mock resignation in his voice as he skimmed the short list of options.

Claire chuckled. "I figured you'd been here before."

Kiernan glanced up from the menu. "To be honest, I've driven by it and admired the flowers, but never stopped in."

"I got to say…you don't strike me as a cucumber sandwich kind of guy."

Kiernan laughed heartily. "Looks like I'm going to have to be today." He perused the limited choices once more. "Or a tomato sandwich guy."

"Let's splurge and get a platter of both."

"Deal."

He placed the menu down and raised a tea toast to Claire, who obliged with a clink of porcelain.

"So, what are some of your favorite spots back home?" Kiernan asked after the waitress had come by to take their order. "There must be an award-winning cucumber sandwich shop back in Boston?"

Claire chuckled. "I'm sure there is. But favorite spots? Hmm… There's a park on the outskirts of the city that I go to whenever I can. It has some nice walking paths. And a pond—with ducks. You might have noticed I really like ducks."

Kiernan laughed as she pondered some more.

"There's also a quirky little bookshop in my town that I really love. It's been family-owned for years—not one of those big chain bookstores. Whenever I go there Marge, one of the owners, will have some hand-picked books put aside for me."

"That sounds wonderful. And what of kind of books do you like to read?"

"Lately, I've been into cozy mysteries."

"Ah, you mean like the little ol' British grandmother who solves crimes while tending to her rose garden?"

Claire snickered. "Sounds like the plot of the last one I read." As Kiernan raised his teacup for another toast, she obliged and said, "Your turn."

"I should have known that was coming…"

"Come on. Favorite places. Spill."

"Well, I think you've already seen both." As Claire raised her eyebrows he added, "The hospital and Gilroy's Pub. Although I guess I should add any rugby field within a sixty-mile radius."

"The hospital is your favorite spot?" she asked curiously.

"Kind of. It's where I spend most of my time."

"All the more reason you need different favorite spots."

"Huh…" Kiernan ruminated on her observation for several moments. "I think I misunderstood the question."

"Nice try."

Kiernan laughed. He was squirming in the hot seat, but just seeing Claire's easy grin was worth the discomfort.

Four finger sandwiches and three cups of sweetened tea later, Kiernan leaned back in his chair and admired the even sweeter view from not so afar. Just across from him, Claire and her serene beauty were nothing short of mesmerizing—and if duty hadn't been calling, he knew he could have got lost in that vision all day. But with a tonsillectomy scheduled for two p.m., he had to get back to the hospital soon.

"Thanks," Kiernan said a few minutes later as the waitress handed him back his bank card. He turned to Claire. "Well, back to the hospital for me—and hopefully back to something enjoyable for you. Have you been doing any fun touristy things?"

"How can I?" Claire replied with a mischievous twinkle in her eye. "You keep interrupting my vacation."

"Ouch." Kiernan chuckled, and when his phone buzzed in his pocket, he was fully prepared to ignore it.

Except medical emergencies had a way of following him.

He pulled out the phone and grimaced. "I'm sorry—this is the hospital."

Silently reading the text message, he felt his jaw and neck instantly tense.

Manchester Gen is out and team confirmed we can't cut thru red tape in time for surgery outside of UK. We're out of options. But wanted to get OK from you before telling Jan.

Kiernan sighed deeply and placed the phone on the table with the screen facing down, unable to pull the trigger that would end Jan's dream of giving birth to a healthy baby.

With a creased forehead and concerned eyes, Claire asked, "Is everything okay?"

"Not really. The last few potential hospitals that could do Jan's surgery in time are no-gos. It looks like we're at the end of the road."

Claire's shoulders dropped, her pale green eyes mirroring the deep disappointment that Kiernan now felt. Silence passed between them, the upbeat atmosphere of a few seconds ago now fully deflated and somber.

Suddenly, a thought sprang into Kiernan's mind. And it was a doozy. As he looked up at Claire she lurched back slightly, as though reverberating with the energy that was bouncing off him.

"I have an idea. A *crazy* idea. But… Okay, just hear me out. If I can get permission from the hospital and make everything else fall into place, would you be able to perform Jan's surgery? The hospital will pay you, of course, and I can't imagine they'd turn down the proposition, knowing how much they want West Mercy to make a name for itself in this sort of surgery. Plus, it would be an amazing experience for my team to learn from someone of your caliber."

Claire appeared stricken as she stared back at him. Her reaction was enough to drop his stomach to his knees.

"Believe me, I know this is a lot to ask." He paused, waiting for her to reply. And waiting some more. "I'm sorry—it was an impulsive thought. I should never have suggested it."

"I... I um...."

Claire's head dropped downwards as she stared at the table. Kiernan didn't need to be a doctor to see that her breathing had accelerated and the color was draining from her face.

Finally, she looked up. "Can I just...? Can I think about it, please? I'll give you an answer by tomorrow. I promise."

"Yes. Yes, of course."

As she started to stand up from the chair, Kiernan stood up as well, quickly stepping over and gently grabbing her arm as she braced her other arm unsteadily against the table. Her skin was soft, but slightly clammy, and as she locked eyes with him, he saw fear bordering on panic. It was the same look he'd seen yesterday.

But why?

Had something happened back at Boston General? Had there been a failed surgery that had been so devastating she'd taken a leave of absence for a month? Not every surgery was successful—no matter how gifted the surgeon. Or perhaps she had become too emotionally involved in a case and the outcome had pushed her over the edge.

Kiernan tightened his jaw, knowing he needed to reel in his suspicions. He was grasping at straws, wanting to understand. But unless she opened up to him, he was blindly guessing at best.

"Thank you for lunch," Claire said. "If I ever crave a mean cucumber sandwich again, I know where to go."

There was a slight quiver in her smile, and the sheer effort to hide her discomfort was almost palpable.

Kiernan watched as Claire headed out of the dining patio, frozen in place until a wave of heightened resolve swept over him. No. *No!* He was *not* going to let her run off like this in such a clearly distressed state of mind. He pulled his phone out of his pocket and waited for the call to be answered.

"Hello, Mr. O'—"

"Lucy," he urgently interjected. "I have a personal matter to attend to and I need you to put Mr. Ramsey on my two p.m. tonsillectomy."

"Yes, I'll let him know right away." There was a brief pause. Then, "Is everything okay?"

He knew why Lucy was asking. If there were two words she had never heard him utter in succession, they were "personal" and "matter."

"Yes," he said, his voice clipped. "I'll touch base with you when I'm back."

Bounding out to the parking lot, he spotted

Claire just as she was about to get into her car. "Claire! Wait!"

She swung around, eyes widened.

She was still holding on to the door handle when he caught up with her. "I can't let you leave like this. Please—can we sit and talk for a bit?"

It took several moments for Claire to find her voice. "I'm not sure what you mean…"

"I've upset you."

"No, I'm fine…really."

Kiernan shook his head. "You're not fine."

Her eyes met his and, surprisingly, she didn't push back on his assessment. He turned and nodded to a cobblestoned path lined with several benches that cut through the flowered grounds.

"Walk with me? Please?"

Perhaps it was the pleading quality to his voice, but Claire slowly closed the car door and together they headed out of the parking lot and onto the path. Several minutes later they were seated on a wooden bench, surrounded by the heady aroma of tulips, daffodils and roses.

"Wait—what about your tonsillectomy?" Claire asked, before Kiernan had a chance to initiate conversation.

"I already called the hospital and another surgeon is filling in for me." He flashed the hint of a smile. "It's one of the advantages of being chief of surgery. I can pass off a procedure to someone else and no one will say anything."

Claire's tense face relaxed slightly as her lips

curved upward. But the smile was short-lived. "If this is about Jan's surgery—your question caught me off guard, that's all."

"I don't care about Jan's surgery," Kiernan replied forcefully. He shook his head and looked briefly up at the sky. "That didn't come out right. Of course I care. But right now my concern is you. I don't mean to pry, Claire, and maybe it's none of my business, but I can't help feeling there's something you're not telling me—something that caused you to react the way you did in the birthing suite yesterday, and now this. Whatever it is, you can talk to me. Maybe I can help. Or I'll just be quiet and listen."

She stared intently into his eyes for what seemed like an eternity, as though debating inwardly whether to open up to him.

"You're right," she said finally. "I haven't been entirely upfront with you as to why I took a leave of absence to come here." She paused, her eyes now glossy and pained. "Seven months ago, I gave birth to a stillborn daughter. Her name was Ariana."

Kiernan flinched, feeling as though an unseen hand had slapped him across the cheek. He had not seen this coming. Not by a longshot. "Claire, I'm so sorry."

Claire blinked several times to push back tears. She started to speak again, but nothing came out.

"You don't have to say any more," Kiernan said quietly.

She took in a deep breath, as if re-energized with

resolve. "I want to. You see, I came to Ireland for a month to figure out if I can continue in my career as an ob-gyn. I know I'm not the first obstetrician to lose a child, and I really thought I would be able to separate my personal pain from my professional life. But I can't. Every time I witness the birth of a healthy baby, I'm glad for the parents, but I also wonder why I didn't have the same happy ending with Ariana. And every miscarriage or stillbirth… it's like reliving her death all over again." Claire's voice cracked, but she pushed herself to finish. "I'm no good to my patients like this. They deserve better. But I just don't know how to get past it all."

Kiernan looked up at the bright afternoon sky, his chest tightening as the unintended repercussions of his actions grew clearer. "And then you come here and right from the start…"

He shook his head, unable to say more. An emergency breech delivery. A consultation on fetal surgery for a serious birth defect. And—the ultimate stab in the heart—being asked to perform complex, high-risk surgery to correct that anomaly in an unborn child. Everything she had been trying to get away from he had been unwittingly throwing her way since her arrival.

"Claire, I'm so sorry that I've caused you pain."

She placed a hand over his, and her soft, warm touch momentarily disrupted his focus.

"None of this is your fault. There was no way you could have known."

So many thoughts and emotions were swirling

around in Kiernan's mind. Not to mention more questions. Such as who and where was Ariana's father? But he wasn't about to ask. The last thing he wanted to do was potentially add salt to a wound whose depths he could not even begin to imagine.

"In case you're wondering, Ariana's father is no longer in the picture."

Kiernan gulped silently. Had Claire just read his mind? "I'm sorry to hear that."

"It's okay. I mean, better to have found out the kind of person he really is now than even further down the road. The CliffsNotes version is that we met in medical school, married after graduation, and he left when I was six months pregnant with Ariana. It turns out he was having an affair with someone at his practice and she recently gave birth to a daughter."

Kiernan narrowed his eyes. "That's despicable."

He wanted to punch the man, surgeon's hands be damned. The satisfaction of inflicting upon him even a fraction of the pain he had caused Claire would be worth a broken knuckle or two.

"Whew!" Claire exclaimed, dabbing at her moistened eyes. "I'm a real joy to be around, huh?"

"You are—and then some," he said quietly, looking into her eyes. "And I never would have asked you to perform Jan's surgery if I had known what you've been going through."

"Believe me, I know that. But my earlier answer hasn't changed. I just need the rest of the day to think everything over."

Kiernan shook his head. "No, I don't think this is a good idea."

Claire squeezed his hand, her reddened eyes offset by a growing smile. "Too late. You already asked me."

Kiernan clenched his jaw as he tried to wrangle a swirl of conflicting emotions. Maybe *he* needed the day to reexamine his thoughts, too. His first instinct was to protect Claire from further pain and trauma. But at the same time she had come to Ireland to determine whether she could reengage in her profession as an ob-gyn. Could successfully performing Jan's surgery, and at a hospital without all the painful memories of Boston General, provide the definitive answer she needed?

He turned to her, nearly overwhelmed by a sudden desire to lean in and kiss her. She stared into his eyes in a way that made him think she, too, might feel the same. And yet he resisted.

Never had he thought twice about seizing the moment when it came to a kiss. But never had anyone revealed something so deeply personal to him. He had sensed from the get-go that Claire was a private person. You weren't going to find her announcing her every thought and action on social media—if you found her there at all. She had made herself vulnerable by sharing with him her loss of Ariana, and he did not take her trust in him lightly. It was a trust he would safeguard at all costs, and the last thing he wanted to do was misconstrue her willingness to open up to him.

Claire briefly looked out over the flowered landscape, a kaleidoscope of colors swaying slightly in the breeze, before turning back to him. "I would imagine you need to get back to the hospital soon."

"I'm in no rush," Kiernan replied—an answer that previously would never have left his lips. This was certainly turning out to be a day of firsts for him.

"Do you mind if we just sit here for a bit?" she asked.

That was an easy question to answer.

"I wouldn't want to be anywhere else."

Claire sat on her now favorite rock by the water as she tossed cracked corn onto the ground. In short order, the chopped golden kernels were gobbled up by the boisterous flock of ducks before her.

Quack-quack-quack. Quack-quack-quack.

"Slow down, guys," she said with an affectionate smile as she tossed more corn their way.

It was a brief respite from the whirlwind of emotions that she was still trying to navigate.

After returning home from the tea shop a half-hour ago, Claire had immediately headed down to the water. Mother Nature had an unfailing way of providing clarity when she needed it most, and today that figurative mother had her work cut out for her.

She had been surprised to receive Kiernan's spur-of-the-moment lunch invite, and even more surprised at how readily she had accepted it. But the reasons had been simple—she'd wanted to see him again, her earlier blinking red caution lights be damned, and it would be an opportunity to make up for her skittish behavior the day before. That objective hadn't gone exactly as planned...but maybe that was good thing.

Claire thought back to a nugget of advice dispensed during one of her post-stillbirth therapy sessions. Holding on to a secret gave it power. And if the secret was a source of pain and grief...well, it would only cause more of the same.

Opening up to Kiernan had profoundly changed something inside of her. She could feel it like a heavy weight lifted not only from her shoulders, but from the deepest corners of her mind. His reaction to her revelation had made it clear that he was fully and unequivocally looking out for her. And though he had pulled back on his suggestion that she perform Jan's surgery, they both knew the stakes. There were no more options left for this mother and her unborn child. She was it.

Claire turned her gaze onto several fluffy yellow ducklings as they waddled close behind their mom. When one lost its balance and tumbled over, the mother turned away from the cracked corn she was just about to devour, and used her beak to nudge him back up.

It was a gesture that grabbed at her heart. But that was what all mothers did, regardless of species. They put their children first. And being part of that beautiful dynamic was one of the reasons she loved being an ob-gyn. Or she had.

Claire stood up from the rock and began walking along the water's edge. Could she get that love back again? It was a question she still couldn't answer—although inside she now felt a fluidity where before there had been only rigidness.

But perhaps she was projecting too far ahead. She could make a difference for Jan and her baby *now*. Kiernan had thrown that opportunity into her lap, and she had to…she *wanted* to…give them every chance for the best outcome possible. And with Kiernan by her side, she could do it.

She cupped a hand over her eyes as the afternoon sun glistened on the water. Slowly, a smile emerged. It was accompanied by a flutter of nerves, but that was okay—big decisions could be disconcerting at first. And the fact that this one came easier—and quicker—than expected only solidified to her that it was the right decision to make.

Claire reached into the pocket of her windbreaker to get her phone, then thought better of it. Knowing Kiernan, if she texted him now instead of in the morning, as planned, he'd think she was jumping the gun.

Knowing Kiernan?

Had she really crossed that invisible line from

regarding him as a professional associate, kept at arm's length, to someone she was beginning to connect with on a much deeper level?

She closed her eyes, knowing very well the answer to that.

Kiernan entered the kitchen of his home and tossed his keys on the counter. He was greeted by silence save for the hum of the refrigerator.

Nothing he could say to himself—certainly not *What a day!* or similar—could come close to sufficing as a recap of the past twelve hours. His spur-of-the-moment lunch with Claire had set off a chain reaction of events and revelations, all of which he was still trying to process.

As his eyes scanned the room—the spotless counters and perfectly lined-up canisters, the sparkling stainless-steel appliances and the neat stack of mail in its designated tray—one word came to mind: *sterile.* Which, if this were an operating theater, would be more than appropriate.

But this was his home, his personal oasis. And suddenly, it all just seemed…strange.

He shook his head, wondering why he had never really noticed this before. Could it be because there was little, if any, distinction between his professional and personal life? That was a *duh* question, he surmised silently.

An image of Claire flashed in his mind, and he wondered what it would be like to come home to the feeling that he had whenever she was near.

It was a feeling that he craved, but one that also scared him. If he gave in to it, then he'd need to reevaluate his whole approach to life—the "must-haves" versus the "can-live-withouts." Full devotion to his career, at the expense of everything else, had always been a must-have. But the more his feelings for Claire were beginning to grow, the more tiny fissures were forming in these notions that had been set in stone.

He'd had a glimpse of one those fissures earlier in the day, when he'd bowed out of performing a surgery so that he could stay with Claire and make sure she was okay. He thought back to the day when his father had passed away. He had been prepping for a coronary artery bypass surgery when he had taken an urgent call from his mother. His father's death from a sudden heart attack had been both unexpected and shocking. But both he and his mother had known the drill all too well. After all, it was his father who had pounded it into him.

Personal matters and relationships came second. *Always.*

And the one thing he had thought that day, as he'd suppressed his emotions and walked into the operating theater without so much as a mention of his loss, feeling the disbelieving eyes of colleagues who had heard the news upon him? *Dad would be proud of me.* Which meant he had been proud of himself.

Only now did he realize how misguided his priorities might have been at that moment.

Realizing he needed some air, Kiernan headed out on the back deck that overlooked the ocean, peering into the darkness. With just a sliver of moonlight, he couldn't see the water, but he could hear every wave that crashed against the cliffs below and smell the brine that brought on an instant head rush.

As a sharp ocean breeze whipped through his hair, Kiernan grabbed the rail of the deck with both hands. He needed to steady himself, because everything around him was churning like a cyclone.

Get a hold of yourself.

He was reeling from Claire's unexpected and deeply personal revelation, and the possibility that she might take on Jan's surgery. That was all this was. *Right?* A lot of raw emotion packed into a short span of time.

Of course, if that was the case, then he'd be on edge every time he came out of a difficult surgery that had been touch-and-go until the final successful moments. He always felt relief for both the patients and their families in those situations, but it had never spurred him to come home and question why the damn refrigerator was the closest thing he had to a significant other after a long day at the hospital.

No, this was about Claire. Of that, he was sure. Seeing her heartache as she'd told him about Ariana...

Could performing Jan's surgery be the catalyst she needed to reengage in her career as an ob-gyn?

The question nearly cut off his air supply, and he took in a deep breath of salty ocean air. He needed to be careful. This was not one medical professional concerned about the career of a peer. For him, at least, it was already so much more. And he couldn't have that in the life he had mapped out for himself.

Unless, of course, he redrew the map.

It was a thought that hit him harder than a tidal wave.

CHAPTER SEVEN

KIERNAN ENTERED THE café on the second floor of the hospital, immediately spotting Claire at a small table in the furthest, most quiet corner. Earlier in the morning she had texted him to say that she wanted to move forward with Jan's surgery, but that alone wasn't enough to convince him. He needed to see her in person, to read her body language and look into her eyes to be certain that *she* was certain.

After all, it was in her nature to want to help others, but he couldn't let that be at the expense of her own well-being.

"Thanks for meeting me here," he said as he sat down next to her.

Dressed in casual jeans and a light pink sweater, she looked downright gorgeous. Then again, Kiernan thought, she could don a burlap sack and still put a designer-clad supermodel to shame. He'd take natural, unfettered beauty over an artificially enhanced appearance any day of the week—and Claire had that in spades.

She smiled, her eyes bright but anxious. "So, you said you wanted to talk to me in person about the surgery. Are you thinking the hospital won't sign off on it?"

"No, that's not why I asked you to come by…" As Claire's smile began to wilt, he knew he couldn't drag out his concerns any longer. "Claire, you don't have to do this."

"I know. But I want to. Look, I don't know what the future holds for me as far as my career goes. I still have a lot to think through. But one thing I know for sure is that I can make a difference for Jan and her baby. And it's the only chance they have at this point. That alone is enough for me to pull it together. I *want* to do this. Besides, we've already proved that we're a pretty good team in an operating room."

Kiernan grinned. "You mean in the back of a bumpy ambulance?"

"Right." She smirked, but then her face grew more serious. "The thing is, after telling you about Ariana…you know my secret now. And somehow… just opening up to you… I feel like it's lessened its hold on me."

Kiernan wanted to believe she was right. For Jan and her baby, yes. But also for Claire's own healing. Her previous reaction in the birthing suite and at yesterday's lunch clearly indicated she was still in the throes of pain and grief over losing Ariana. Could sharing her loss really have changed all that? Silently, he tossed the question around in his mind, his face tense with concern.

"What's wrong?" Claire asked, picking up on his doubts.

"I'm just worried that you might not be ready to

take on this surgery. You've been through so much. How do you know you won't be triggered by something that happens in Theater? I'm afraid it might be too much, too soon."

"Believe me, I've thought about this. I'd never put Jan and her baby at risk. I'm not going into this surgery thinking it will help me decide once and for all what to do about my career. That would be putting too much pressure on myself. But I do know that right here, right now, I'm fully committed to doing everything I can to help them. And knowing you'll be with me in the operating room…"

Her voice trailed off, but Kiernan knew what she was implying—that his presence would have a stabilizing effect on her should a potential trigger arise. He wanted to believe that was true, but wasn't entirely sold on the notion.

Once again, Claire seemed to home in on his doubts.

"You know how people sometimes hold a paper clip when they're giving a speech to calm their nerves? Well, you'll be my paper clip in the operating room."

He raised an amused eyebrow. "You mean like a surgical lucky charm?"

It wasn't his intention to make light of a serious situation, only to help put her at ease. And himself, too, for that matter.

"Something like that, yes." She snickered slightly, then grew more serious. "So, given that Jan's surgery needs to happen very soon, we do need to go over some specifics. I'm sure you already know this, but this is an all hands on deck procedure. I'll need every specialist in every discipline that you've got. Cardiology, neurology, pediatrics—and they'll need to get up to speed on the surgery itself. I mean, is all of that even possible on such short notice?"

"I'll *make* it possible," Kiernan replied, pulling confidence out of thin air given all that needed to fall into place—and fast. "I'm going to call an emergency meeting with the board. It's probably too short notice to get everyone together today, but I should be able to set something up for first thing tomorrow morning. And I'll have my surgery co-ordinator get to work on putting together a comprehensive team."

"Will you wait to get the okay before telling Jan?"

"I think that would be best. The last thing I want to do is falsely get her hopes up. I don't think there'll be any major roadblocks to moving forward with the surgery, but best to be sure first."

Claire nodded, her face visibly relaxing. "Good."

"So, now that that's settled, I have some doctor's orders for you."

She raised an eyebrow. "Oh?"

Kiernan extracted a prescription pad from the pocket of his white coat, scribbled away for a few moments, then tore off a piece of paper and handed it to her.

Claire twisted her mouth to one side with amusement before reading it out loud: "'*You are to spend*

*the next twenty-four hours playing with ducks,
reading a cozy mystery, exploring a castle and eating cucumber sandwiches to your heart's desire.
Unlimited refills.'"*

"Don't be one of those patients who refuses to
take good advice," Kiernan said with a twinkle in
his eyes.

Claire laughed. "I'll do my best."

Claire tapped her fingers on the black-lacquered
chair-arm and stared at the TV screen in front of
her. A football game was in full swing, and though
the half-dozen other occupants in the room sat
glued to the action, her eyes—and thoughts—wandered as she waited in vain for time to speed up.

More than twenty-four hours had passed since
she had met with Kiernan in the café and, like a
partially dutiful patient, she had played with the
ducks and toured a local castle. But the cozy mystery book would have to wait. And the cucumber
sandwiches…? Those would have to wait, too. Perhaps indefinitely….

With a silent sigh, she once again glanced at the
large digital clock on the adjacent wall of one of
West Mercy's smaller waiting rooms. The original
plan had been for Kiernan to call her as soon as the
board meeting ended, but sitting at the cottage to
await such a pivotal decision had made her so antsy
that she'd been ready to go search for a sand hill.

Instead, she had texted Kiernan to say that she
was on her way to the hospital so that she could

hear the good news in person. Of course, that presumed that there would *be* good news. But she had to hold on to hope.

Suddenly, she caught a flash of movement out of the corner of her eye. Kiernan swept into the waiting room, his commanding presence prompting those around her to instinctively sit up straighter in their chairs. His serious face was devoid of a smile, and Claire's shoulders sank as her own smile faded in response.

And then a thumb shot up as a Cheshire cat grin spread from ear to ear. "We're on," he said as Claire sprang from her chair.

She caught herself just short of pouncing on him with hug-ready arms. Clearing her throat, she tucked several loose locks of hair behind her ear, dropped her arms woodenly to her sides, and said, in a measured, low-key voice, "That's fantastic news."

Kiernan was still viewing her through widened eyes, as though he was fully prepared for and looking forward to being tackled, and seemed disappointed that she'd reversed course at the last second.

"Did you get any pushback?" Claire asked, hoping the inquiry would erase the awkward moment she had created between them.

"They had a lot of questions, of course. And there are still some logistics to work out. But they also understand that time is of the essence. They're looking at it as a major milestone for West Mercy.

But I think you'll agree with me that the biggest win is for Jan and her baby."

"Absolutely. When do you plan to tell her?"

"*We* can tell her right now. She had a follow-up ultrasound appointment today, and I told the technician to let her know that I wanted to touch base with her before she left. I wasn't sure we'd have good news to share, but I hedged my bets and now we actually do."

Twenty minutes later, Claire and Kiernan exited the consultation room after sharing the good news with Jan. As expected, she was equal parts ecstatic and nervous—a completely normal reaction in the face of surgery that held the highest hopes for her unborn baby, yet was far from routine and simple.

At one point, Jan had shared the fact that she and her husband had decided to learn the sex of the baby, and had named their daughter Rhianna. The similar ring to Ariana had caught Claire by surprise, but one glance in Kiernan's direction, his expression both knowing and understanding, and she had quickly been pulled back to the present. That she could acknowledge her pain without being instantly transported back to a very dark place was testament to the healing power of sharing her secret. And not with just anyone, of course, but with Kiernan, whom she was trusting more and more.

As they continued down the corridor a flurry of thoughts vied for Claire's attention. She always felt as though she was balancing on a tightrope when reassuring patients about the outcome of a complex surgery. She believed in her skills, and all of her previous spina bifida fetal surgeries to date had been successful. But that didn't mean complications couldn't arise. And to be performing this procedure at an unfamiliar hospital, with an inexperienced team as far as fetal surgery was concerned... Well, she'd have to be in deep denial not to realize the risk factor was far from non-existent.

"I know it's a lot of pressure to perform this surgery under such unusual circumstances," Kiernan said, perhaps picking up on her concern. "But I want to assure you that we're doing everything at our end to be fully prepared by Monday. You said this is an all hands on deck situation, and I have nearly two dozen surgeons and specialists coming in this weekend to go over everything ahead of time. They might not all need to be present for the surgery on Monday, but we're covering all ground just in case."

"I should be there," Claire said, wondering why she hadn't thought to offer before.

"I don't think that will be necessary. You came to Ireland to get away from it all, and I don't want you to be pulled back into the medical world any more than necessary."

"I think it's a little too late for that," Claire said, with a touch of humor in her voice.

Kiernan half grinned. "I know. But I've found some great training videos from the hospital that pioneered this procedure, and they're about as thorough as you can get. We'll all study everything over the weekend, and on Monday we'll get an early start so you can address the team and take any last-minute questions. If something comes up during the training this weekend that requires your input, I'll give you a call." He slowed his pace and turned to her. "Does that sound like a plan?"

She smiled. "Yes, that sounds like a plan."

Suddenly, he came to a halt. "Actually, there *is* a bit of bad news that I should have mentioned earlier."

Claire felt her stomach sink.

"The board is haggling about appropriate payment for the surgery and, knowing how slow this sort of thing moves through the system, I think it might be another week or two before the money can be transferred to you."

Claire breathed a sigh of relief. "Oh—that! I should have mentioned this earlier as well. I'm not looking to get paid for the surgery."

Kiernan nearly balked. "That's hugely generous of you, but I can't let you perform such a time-intensive, complex surgery for free. Let the hospital cough something up to compensate you fairly—as well they should."

"How about you let them figure out what they think my services are worth, and whatever it is, I'll donate it to a worthy cause. You can choose what that should be, since I'm not familiar with local organizations. But maybe something like a women's shelter, or a women's health educational program?"

Kiernan stared at her in near-disbelief. "Have I told you lately that you're amazing?"

Claire felt her face flush, and an appreciative smile was the only reply she could manage.

They resumed walking, but took only a few steps before Kiernan stopped and turned to her. "Actually, if you're not going to accept payment, then I have a counteroffer."

"Which is…?" Claire asked, equal parts cautious and intrigued.

"Let me cook dinner for you tomorrow night at my place."

Claire gulped silently. "Dinner?" Another silent gulp. "At your place?"

"It's not a dungeon, I swear," Kiernan replied, prompting a slightly nervous smile from Claire. "Plus, remember how I failed at your question about my favorite spots?"

"Miserably, as I recall."

Kiernan grinned. "Well, this is a chance for me to amend my answer. I have an outdoor deck that virtually dangles over the cliffs and looks out onto the ocean. I might be biased, but it's one of the most magnificent views on the West Coast of Ireland."

Claire grimaced apprehensively. "'Dangles over the cliffs'? You need to work on your sales pitch."

Kiernan laughed. "It's one hundred percent safe and secure, I promise."

"Mr. O'Rourke! Mr. O'Rourke!"

Kiernan and Claire turned in the direction of the eager voice, watching as a young boy ran toward them while his mother tried to keep pace close behind.

"Henry!" Kiernan exclaimed, returning the boy's high five before giving his carrot-red hair an affectionate tousle. "What a wonderful surprise!" He looked up at the boy's mother. "Catherine, how are you?"

"Hello, Mr. O'Rourke. I'm doing great." She smiled from ear to ear. "And, more importantly, *Henry's* doing great."

"I'm on the school rugby team now!" Henry exclaimed.

Kiernan's eyes widened. "Fantastic! What position?"

"Inside center—just like you."

"Best position there is," Kiernan said with a wink.

He turned to Claire and commenced introductions, summing up his history with Henry as being one of many West Mercy doctors who'd banded together to treat the young boy after a life-threatening car accident four years ago.

"Mr. O'Rourke is being far too modest," Catherine said to Claire. "He headed up a team that not only saved Henry's life, but saved his leg—which at one point wasn't a certainty." She looked down at her son, beaming with pride. "And now he's playing rugby on the school team. If that's not a miracle, I don't know what is."

"Were you in today for a recheck?" Kiernan asked.

Catherine nodded. "We had an annual appointment with Mr. O'Leary to make sure everything is working as it should with Henry's leg. Although after Henry bounded into the room and more or less catapulted himself onto the table, Mr. O'Leary said he probably doesn't need to see him again—at least not in an official capacity."

"With an entrance like that, who needs X-rays, right?" Kiernan observed to all-around laughter.

Claire discreetly stepped back. Not only to give Kiernan and Henry some room for their boisterous reunion, but also to make sure her eyes—and ears—weren't playing tricks on her. Because if she hadn't known better, she'd have thought Kiernan—he of the "I don't see children in my future" mantra—was carrying on in a downright paternal manner. Which meant that suddenly, and quite unexpectedly, she could see him as a father. And not just as *any* father, but the kind she would want for her own children.

Whoa, whoa, whoa!

Claire took another step back—but this time because she had just jumped so far out in front of herself. In the span of a few seconds she'd started to see Kiernan in a whole new light—one that made him even more attractive than before, if that was possible. And for the first time since losing Ariana, the thought of having another child had entered her mind.

"Claire?"

Claire jerked her head up just in time to see Henry and his mother departing down the corridor.

"They said goodbye to you, but I don't think you heard them."

Slightly dazed, Claire steadied herself and smiled. "Sorry, I…um… I got distracted."

He cocked his head to one side. "You okay?"

"Yes." Another smile…this time with less effort needed.

"Good. Well, before you head out let's settle on a time for dinner tomorrow. How about if I pick you about seven p.m.?" As Claire's eyes widened, he added, "I know…you love your Mini. But my place is rather remote and tricky to find, and this will just make it easier."

She allowed herself to breathe again. "Yes, of course. That makes sense."

As Claire walked through the parking lot to her car, a short time later, she tried to wrap her head around the dizzying speed at which everything seemed to be swirling around her. Hadn't she come to Ireland to slow things down and mull over her future? Instead, she was about to dive headfirst back into the high-stakes medical world that she had put on hold. And, even more confounding, although romance had been the last thing on her mind when she'd arrived here, the universe seemed to have other ideas.

How else to explain why someone like Kiernan had almost instantly landed in the midst of everything and every moment spent with him since had been nothing short of magical?

Cupping her hand over her eyes, she looked up at the bright sky, quietly saying out loud, "You're either one very smart universe…" She paused, knowing full well that her time with Kiernan was limited. "Or the joke's on me."

CHAPTER EIGHT

CLAIRE TOOK ONE final look at her reflection in the bathroom mirror, sighed deeply, then headed to the main room in her cottage to wait for Kiernan. The fact that she had changed her outfit three times, segued from a hair-twist to a sleek ponytail and finally loose tresses, told her one thing.

This is not good.

Her attraction to Kiernan had gone beyond the point where she could convince herself that it was simply admiration for his surgical prowess. There was the way he'd been so understanding when she'd opened up to him about Ariana. His supportive concern about her own well-being if she were to perform Jan's high-stakes surgery, which in turn had infused her with the courage she needed to step back into the world of obstetrics.

And can we talk about that thick, run-your-fingers-through-it dark hair and that muscular rugby build?

Claire took a deep breath and reminded herself that this wasn't a date...or was it? Kiernan might have tried to frame the dinner as a substitute payment for her doing the surgery, but she'd have been remiss not to have seen the anticipation in his eyes when he'd made the offer. Especially since it had matched her own.

Just be yourself.

That was all she could do, right? Real date or sort-of date—this was still the first date of *any* kind since her marriage to Mark had ended. And that alone had her alternating between nervousness and excitement.

A knock at the door brought Claire's racing thoughts to a halt. At least temporarily. They came flooding back as soon as she opened the door.

It should have dawned on her that any man who was a feast for the eyes in drab scrubs would be impossible to look away from in dressier clothes. Which in this case were crisp jeans and a light gray casual sports coat over a form-fitting black T-shirt. Mouth slightly agape, her mind drew a blank as it searched for a standard greeting.

Kiernan smiled, and as his lips curved upwards, her knees buckled downwards. "Hi."

Oh, that's the word.

"Hi," she replied.

"You look beautiful."

"So do you."

As they shared a laugh at her awkward comment, Claire inwardly admonished herself.

Don't be a dork. Please.

A short time later she was seated in the passenger seat of Kiernan's silver hybrid SUV as it effortlessly climbed a steep, winding road framed on both sides by lush green fields.

"I guess you weren't kidding about living in a remote area," Claire observed five more miles into the journey, as the off-the-grid scenery grew increasingly breathtaking.

He turned to her and grinned. "It gets even better."

When she stepped out of the SUV fifteen minutes later, it was with a sense of awe. She walked with Kiernan up the short driveway and viewed the modern, eco-friendly dwelling before her. With more glass than solid walls, its presence was considerable, despite its relatively modest size.

"I was expecting a stone cottage, but this is... wow."

"Thanks. I fell in love with this spot, but there weren't any existing homes. So I bought a parcel of land and had this one built five years ago."

Once inside, Kiernan commenced a brief tour, and Claire couldn't help but notice the tidy, everything-in-its-place décor. She was about to ask jokingly if he sterilized his eating utensils with the same autoclaving method of surgical instrument sanitization, when she spotted a vase of vibrant blue flowers on the kitchen counter that could easily double as a "what doesn't belong here?" picture riddle.

"They're beautiful," she said as she leaned over to smell them. "Did you pick them yourself?"

"I did—from the side of a cliff."

Claire did a double-take. "I never realized flower-gathering could be such a high-risk endeavor."

Kiernan smiled, and when he answered there was a tinge of pride in his voice. "Nothing that some spiked shoes and a sturdy rope couldn't solve. I thought you might like them. It was either the flowers or some ducks, and I figured the flowers would be easier to maintain indoors."

Claire laughed, touched that he'd gone to such extremes on her behalf. She didn't want to read *too* much into the gesture…but it was hard not to conclude that he wouldn't have done this for just anyone.

"Let's head outside."

Kiernan led Claire out to the cedar deck attached to the back of the house.

"Holy moly, Kiernan! This view is unbelievable," Claire said breathlessly as she looked out onto the ocean. "I can see why it's a favorite spot."

"Just don't look down."

"Too late," Claire said as she grasped the deck railing with both hands. "You really *are* dangling off a cliff!"

"More like a highly engineered teetering," Kiernan observed wryly as he opened the bottle of wine that rested in the center of a wrought-iron table, complete with two fancy place settings. He then joined Claire, and together they leaned their folded arms on the railing and looked out onto the waves as they crashed against the cliff.

"Is the water always this turbulent?" Claire asked curiously.

Kiernan nodded. "Enough so that on the rare

day when things are relatively still, I start to worry that there's an earthquake or something in store."

They silently appreciated the view for another minute, then Kiernan turned to her.

"I hope you're hungry?"

"That depends on how good the chef is," Claire teased.

"I'll have you know my deep-dish, three-cheese lasagna has been a hit at every West Mercy staff summer picnic for the past six years."

"I'm impressed. So what's on the menu tonight?"

Kiernan's left cheek creased with a one-sided smile. "Deep-dish, three-cheese lasagna."

Claire chuckled. "Ah, so you're a one-trick pony?"

"I beg your pardon?" Kiernan replied, feigning insult. "More like a prize steed that knows enough to stick to a winning formula."

Claire laughed.

"I thought we could dine out here."

Kiernan walked over to a stone-encased fire pit and lit the aromatic wood inside. As if on cue, the string of dusk-to-dawn automatic lights that spanned the surrounding deck rail blinked on.

"Look at this..." Claire scanned the softly glowing deck. "It's like Gilroy's Pub after dark—minus the drunken rugby players and the smell of stale beer."

"My teammates are just a phone call away if you'd prefer the full Gilroy's experience."

Claire grinned. "Thanks, I'm good."

"I was hoping you'd say that." Kiernan pulled out a chair at the table and waited for Claire to be seated. "I was looking forward to dinner just the two of us."

Claire wondered if Kiernan could actually hear her gulp.

Yup, I think this is a date.

With considerable effort, she corralled the butterflies in her stomach that had been set off by a rush of adrenaline.

Just go with the flow, she reminded herself, though it was easier said than done.

"I'm going to go check on my fan favorite lasagna. Be back in a minute."

Claire nodded and smiled. He could serve her a baked hockey puck and she'd probably think it was a culinary masterpiece. Not that he needed to know that, of course.

Twenty minutes later, Claire placed her fork and knife together on her empty plate and pushed it slightly forward, more than pleasantly surprised. "That was delicious. My compliments to the chef."

"You mean the one-trick pony?"

Claire grinned. "All joking aside, you're a great cook. I'm surprised."

Kiernan pretended to choke on her comment. "I'm not *too* insulted."

"Ha! I just mean I'm surprised you find the time to cook with your schedule."

"You did catch the part where I told you I have one recipe in my arsenal, right?"

"Well, it's a winner."

"Glad it wasn't awful. More wine?"

"Please."

Her glass replenished, she glanced over at the fire pit, her eyes lingering on the dancing flames for longer than she had intended. Perhaps because they were a metaphor for the question that was burning inside of her. She turned back to Kiernan. Dare she ask him? A few more seconds of contemplation, and then impulse took over.

"So, I'm curious about something…" she began.

Kiernan cocked his head slightly to one side. "Go on."

"At the hospital yesterday, when you were talking with Henry, I couldn't help but notice how… natural…you were around him. In fact, if I didn't know any better, I'd say you actually *like* children."

Kiernan's expression changed from one of intrigue to confusion. "I *do* like children. What makes you think I don't?"

"Well, you said before that you don't want children."

"I said I don't think I can fully devote myself to my career and children at the same time. One or the other would have to give. It's just the way it is. And my decision to put my career first has nothing to do with any imagined prestige of being chief of surgery. It's that I get to save lives. I mean, *you* know what that feeling is like. It's a huge responsibility and one that I don't take lightly. And it's because I *do* like children that I'd never subject them to the type of childhood I had with an absentee father."

Claire managed a faint nod. "I get it."

She could leave it at that. She *should* leave it at that. Except...

"But on the other hand, I can think of a number of colleagues back home—both men and women—who are very involved with their children and are still top-notch doctors who give one hundred percent to their patients."

Kiernan pursed his lips together and stared at Claire, as though trying to discern why she was grilling him on this matter. "I don't know," he finally replied. "Maybe some doctors can strike that perfect balance. I suppose it depends what field of medicine they're in. Some are more demanding than others." He paused. "And I've never shied away from admitting my views have been shaped in large part by the fact that my father was a very dedicated surgeon, but an incredibly inattentive father."

"And that realization isn't enough to make you wonder if there might be another way?"

As soon as the question left Claire's mouth, she knew she had to stop. She was pushing Kiernan too far—raising questions that might be appropriate if they had just embarked on a relationship, but not as very temporary colleagues. It didn't matter if there was a part of her that yearned for more with him.

Did I just admit that?

It was not something that could ever be. Soon,

there would be three thousand miles between them. And did she really need to remind herself about their conflicting views on parenthood yet again?

She could see in Kiernan's eyes that he was struggling to form an answer to her question. So she decided to make it easy for him. Perhaps for them both.

"I don't think we've had an official toast yet." She raised her glass of wine. "Here's to a successful surgery for Jan and Rhianna."

Kiernan's tense face softened, and he raised his glass as well. "I will happily drink to that."

Claire smiled, then took a sip of wine. It was a mellow Merlot that initially tasted sweet on her lips, but quickly morphed into bitterness. Funny how it mirrored her growing feelings for Kiernan, she thought. A dream that was so enticing, and a reality that cut like a knife.

"Hard to believe I'm halfway through my stay here," she said pensively.

Kiernan's smile was cut short, though it soon re-emerged with what appeared to be some effort. "It seems like just yesterday we were strangers who met on a hillside during a medical crisis," he said.

"It does…" An uncomfortable silence filled the air, and Claire scrambled to break its hold. "So, I guess I have some catching up to do if I'm going to play tourist for the remainder of my time here. Any suggestions?"

Kiernan's face instantly lit up. "What you really

need is a good tourist guide. Someone who knows Ireland like the back of his hand."

"Hmm… Do you have anyone in mind?"

"I do. He's a great conversationalist and he knows all the hidden gems that the big tour companies miss. Plus, I heard that for certain individuals— make that certain *very special* individuals—his services are free."

Claire had been gamely playing along with what she assumed was a playful ruse until she saw the look of earnestness on Kiernan's face. "Wait, you're not serious…are you?"

"That I'm a great conversationalist? Gift of the Blarney here. I just happen to hide it well." He winked. "At least when I'm in surgeon mode."

"But how are you going to get time off from the hospital on such short notice?"

"Leave that up to me. I probably have about five years' worth of unused leave at this point."

"Why do I not find that hard to believe?"

Kiernan smirked. "So, what do you say?"

"Surgeon, restaurateur and now tour guide. You're quite the entrepreneur."

"The day I announce I'm a sheep herder, too— that's when you have to start worrying."

Claire snickered. "Duly noted."

She paused, grappling with a modified version of an angel on one shoulder, a devil on the other. In this instance it consisted of an angel on each side. On the left shoulder, the angel advised her to let down her protective guard and follow her heart.

And on the right? Well, that angel had something to say about her heart, too.

This situation can't go anywhere. You'll only be hurt.

Both angels were looking out for her. But though she typically erred on the side of caution—especially with matters of the heart—in this moment, and with this man, she was willing to plunge into the unknown, consequences be damned.

She took a deep breath, silently acknowledging that such a cavalier attitude could come back to bite her. But Kiernan was both smart and perceptive. He had to know as well as she did that there was no future for them beyond the next two weeks. Perhaps he *did* just want to show her some interesting sights off the beaten path. There was no harm in that…right?

"So, when does my personalized tour begin?" Claire asked, her voice a tad too flirty for her own liking. "Given that we first have a very major surgery to get through on Monday."

Kiernan pulled his phone out of his pants pocket and scrolled through his calendar. "How does Tuesday sound? I have a carotid endarterectomy in the morning, and an afternoon of administrative work that I'll be more than happy to push to another day."

"Tuesday works. And is there a particular dress code for whatever you have in store?"

As thoughts of a bare-chested Kiernan in an Irish kilt flooded her mind—a most enticing dress code for *him*—she did her best to keep her eyes from popping out of her head.

"Well, I know you like being outdoors—especially when there are ducks around." As Claire laughed, he added, "So let's plan on a countryside walkabout. I have just the place in mind."

"I'll toast to that," she said, clinking her wine glass against his.

She took a sip and swallowed it down, doing her best to shut out the inner whispers of warning from the angel on her right shoulder.

It was that very same shoulder that Kiernan looked past as he pointed behind her. "The moon's just starting to come up. This is the best time of the night—when it's still partially dusk and the light of the moon hits the water." He stood up and offered his hand. "Let's go take a look."

Claire's breath caught in her throat as he took her hand and helped her up from the chair. As he stared into her eyes she felt as though she might melt into the deck boards. Even the brief stroll to the railing felt like a dream. Had she walked there, or floated? She couldn't be sure…

As they leaned over the railing and looked down onto the foamy waves that shimmered with moonlight, a strong breeze came up from the ocean, whipping Claire's hair around her face and shoulders.

"It's chilly, isn't it?" Kiernan asked, turning to her.

In the diminishing light of dusk, his normally

light brown eyes were a shade of dark espresso, but the kindness behind them was unaltered.

Claire crossed her arms tightly in front of her. "Woo! It's like a twenty-degree temperature-drop here."

Wrapping his arm around her side, Kiernan pulled her in close, the warmth of his muscular body seeping into her skin. Now she was *really* melting into the ground… And as he looked into her eyes, she knew he wanted to kiss her. And she wanted to kiss him, too.

He brushed a wayward lock of hair from her cheek, moving his face closer to hers…closer… closer…and then he stopped.

Claire held her breath for several moments. A kiss hadn't passed between them, but in those last seconds, as their eyes locked, an understanding had. Because even though she couldn't imagine a more perfect and atmospheric backdrop to her first kiss with Kiernan, this wasn't the right time.

Her attraction to him was growing exponentially and, as such, it was occupying a huge space in her thoughts and emotions. But right now that space needed to be devoted to one thing above all else: walking back into an operating room on Monday, a path still strewn with trauma from the past, and successfully completing a complex surgery that might also help decide the fate of her career.

And after the surgery? Hopefully there would still be time to pick up where they had just left off.

But with her return to Boston imminent, that time was ticking by fast.

No wonder the angel on her right shoulder was whispering in her ear: *Don't get too attached, Claire.*

One, two, three, four, five... Er...yeah, I think that makes six...

Later that night, with his eyes closed, Kiernan counted the number of opportunities he had had over the course of the evening to take Claire into his arms and kiss her. Fully. Passionately. Deeply. There were probably some more adjectives he could add into the mix, but three was enough to get the point across.

He was able to recall each instance with vivid detail, as though they were playing out in real time in his mind.

Leaning closely over her shoulder as he poured her another glass of wine.

Taking her hand and helping her up from her chair.

Standing side by side at the deck railing after dinner as they gazed out into the moonlit sky—*ugh, I really blew that one*—the waves crashing below them.

Walking her up to her cottage door at the end of the evening to make sure she got safely inside.

And not even then?

Truth be told, he couldn't recall ever struggling to get up the nerve to kiss someone when the circumstances seemed right. But the situation with Claire was different. And the reason was simple, really. He didn't want to scare Claire off before he had a chance to show her…well, *what?* That he was the perfect man for her, despite the fact that they lived thousands of miles apart and had incompatible views on children?

And then there was the matter of Monday's surgery. The last thing he'd wanted to do was to complicate things by throwing a kiss into the mix. There was so much riding on this procedure. For Jan and Rhianna, of course. But for Claire as well. In fact, her very future as an ob-gyn might depend on how everything turned out. Which meant it was imperative that extra distractions be barred from the operating room.

Keep it professional.

At least until after the surgery. And then, if he got the chance to kiss her again— No, wait… *When* he got the chance to kiss her again, he would make up for lost time.

Time. That was another complicating factor that he had to push from his mind. Soon—make that *very* soon—Claire would be heading back to the States for good. And his earlier resolve to just enjoy the now?

What had initially been a *problem solved* solution, was now one that filled him with a growing sense of unease.

CHAPTER NINE

CLAIRE'S PHONE ALARM went off at precisely four a.m. on Monday, as planned, but she was already awake, eyes fixated on the dark ceiling above her. Today, she would be altering the course of life for a mother and her unborn child. She wouldn't blame anyone for thinking she was full of herself to reach such a heady conclusion, but it was true. And it had nothing to do with a biased self-assessment of her skills. If everything went as planned, Rhianna would have as normal a life as possible for a child with a spina bifida birth defect. She had seen—and been the catalyst for—such miracles firsthand in the past.

But if complications arose....

Claire sat up in bed and rested on her elbows for several moments. She wasn't going to go there. Only positive thoughts. She was a firm believer that they could make a difference in the operating room and in life in general. But sometimes, in the latter instance, it was easier said than done—especially in light of personal loss.

But today wasn't about her. It was about Jan and Rhianna, about Jan's husband Dave, and their other two children, Melody and Sean. She had to be strong for them.

Claire reminded herself that Kiernan would be by her side throughout the procedure and instantly felt calmer. He had texted her several times to check in and let her know that the weekend-long intense training session with his team had gone well. They were ready to go. And so was she.

The sun was just beginning to rise as she pulled into the West Mercy staff parking lot. The security guards knew to expect her arrival, and ushered her in after viewing her Boston General photo ID. From the side entrance, it was a three-minute walk to the new neonatal wing, but with the weight of what lay ahead, it felt more like thirty.

After Ariana's death, walking to the OR for a scheduled surgery had felt like trudging through a black cloud. But now? She felt a fluttering of nerves mixed with the anticipated joy and relief of a successful outcome. An unsuccessful outcome, and that black cloud would be back and ten times thicker.

Think only good thoughts, Claire inwardly reminded herself. *Just be fully in the moment for Jan and Rhianna.*

Kiernan and a handful of his colleagues were conversing by the nurses' station as she entered the wing. He turned to her as she approached the group and she quietly caught her breath. Could everyone see how she was looking at him not only as a fellow doctor, but also as the man whose desirable lips had nearly touched her own several nights ago?

She hoped not. Just because *she* had thought about that near-kiss all weekend long, it didn't mean anyone else—other than Kiernan, of course—had any inkling of their dinner together. And she preferred it to stay that way. Effectively leading a new team through a complex surgery required being seen as a top-notch professional in their eyes. And fantasizing about locking lips with the hunky chief of surgery didn't exactly cater to that image.

"Good morning, Dr. Delaney."

The smile on Kiernan's face seemed overly calm—and also quite familiar. It was the "pre-surgery smile" that Claire had come to perfect herself over the years, an almost Zen-like state of mind that descended upon her as she readied for a grueling surgery. The only difference was that his smile was accompanied by a twinkle in his eye. Perhaps he was reminiscing about their almost-kiss, too?

Turning back to the small group, Kiernan said, "If you'll excuse me for a few minutes," then gestured to Claire to follow him.

After a short walk down the hall, he opened a door and peered inside, then switched on the lights. Once they were both inside, he closed the door and turned his full attention on Claire.

"How are you feeling?" he asked, eyes gazing steadily into hers.

Over the years, she had been privy to countless one-on-one interactions with fellow doctors in the privacy of a hospital room or staff quarters…and none had ever made her feel weak in the knees like she did at this moment.

It's pre-surgery jitters, that's all.

If ever she'd needed that Zen mindset, it was now. There was so much riding on this surgery—the most obvious being the best possible outcome for Jan and Rhianna. But there was much at stake on a personal level as well. She needed to stay one hundred percent objective before, during and immediately after the complex procedure—a feat that was easier said than done. Letting even a tiny fraction of her personal pain and angst seep into her performance in the operating room could have devastating consequences.

Would she be able to keep a tight lid on her emotions? She wouldn't have agreed to take on the surgery if she hadn't believed that she could. But now that the moment of reckoning was imminent….

"Claire?"

Kiernan's voice cut into her thoughts, and not a moment too soon. It was time to focus on one thing and one thing only: a successful fetal surgery.

"Sorry," she finally managed to say. "I'm okay. Just giving myself an inner pep talk, that's all."

"You've got this, Claire. I know you do."

He reached over and clasped both her hands. His hands were warm and strong, and his touch sent her brain and body to places that they didn't need to go right now.

"You're going to come through this with flying colors. And you know why?"

Claire was too breathless to answer.

"Because once you do, a special outing awaits with a devastatingly handsome surgeon from West Mercy who moonlights as a tour guide. Or so I've heard…"

In an instant, Claire's flailing nerves were flattened on the spot, and she shook her head and grinned. "I'll keep that in mind."

He squeezed her hands tighter. "All kidding aside, I know how strong you are. But I know this surgery is bringing up a lot of personal issues for you as well. Let's just get in that operating theater and give Jan and Rhianna the happy ending they deserve. Then we'll deal with the other stuff."

We? Did he say "we"?

Claire swallowed hard, reminding herself that now was not the time to read too much into anything that Kiernan might say. He was merely helping her double down on her earlier silent pep talk, and for that she was grateful.

Her resolve now cemented, she looked back up into Kiernan's eyes. "Let's do this."

He smiled and slowly let go of her hands, as though reluctant to break the connection, then opened the door and held it for her to pass through.

There was no turning back now.

As promised, Kiernan assembled the large team just outside the OR for a pre-surgery pep talk. With all eyes focused on her—eager eyes, at that—there was little that Claire needed to say. It was clear that everyone understood the gravity of the situation, but also the miraculous possibilities. And they would all be part of that miracle now.

Once in the OR, Jan was wheeled in, groggy from the IV anesthesia medication that had been started in the pre-surgery area, but still cognizant enough to squeeze Claire's hand as she assured her that they were going to take good care of her and Rhianna.

Sebastian placed a face mask over Jan's nose and mouth, administering the gases that would send her into a deep sedation.

Scalpel in hand, Claire briefly looked up at Kiernan where he stood directly across the operating table. With his surgical mask in place, she could only see his eyes, but they spoke volumes.

You can do this. And I'm right here with you.

She waited as one of the OR nurses swabbed Jan's belly with antiseptic, then performed a laparotomy across her abdomen. With Jan's uterus exposed, Dr. Fleming moved in and began performing an ultrasound to determine Rhianna's position. All eyes were on the ultrasound monitor as her tiny body came into view.

"We'll need to rotate her slightly to gain full access to the spinal opening," Claire said, carefully but firmly placing her gloved hands on each side of Rhianna's body and exerting pressure on the left. This prompted Rhianna to roll slightly to the right—enough of a shift to reposition her spinal opening.

Claire looked to her left at Dr. Fleming who, without needing to be asked, stepped over to confirm the repositioning through ultrasound. This seamless communication—with no actual words needed—was so important in a surgery such as this, with so many moving parts, and Claire appreciated the doctor's diligence.

"Perfect," Claire said quietly as she viewed the spinal defect on the monitor, in the exact spot where it needed to be.

A surgical nurse handed her a uterine stapling device.

"You did a great job prepping your team," Claire said as she looked up at Kiernan.

"We had a very productive weekend," he said. "Saturday was chock-full of training videos, and Sunday was a simulated run-through of the surgery. Make that *many* run-throughs."

"It shows."

She nodded her appreciation in every direction, her eyes creased at the corners as her hidden lips curved upwards. Every doctor who had ever donned a surgical mask knew that this was the OR equivalent of a smile. But there was one doctor in particular whose silent encouragement she needed most. Looking across the operating table, she locked eyes with Kiernan and held his gaze for several moments. The exchange was silent, but the message was the same.

You can do this. I'm right here with you.

After a slight nod of acknowledgement, Claire took a deep breath, then cut into Jan's uterus with the stapling device. She flipped the attachment arm of her microscope glasses downward, instantly revealing a detailed closeup of the myelomeningocele sac, a thin, bluish, fluid-containing membrane about an inch and a half long that protruded from the opening in Rhianna's back.

Here we go.

Her breathing calm and her hands steady, she carefully excised the sac and placed it into a pan. A critical part of the surgery was now complete, but the time-intensive delicate closing of the spinal opening remained. Knowing that this multi-layer closing was normally performed in tandem by a fetal surgeon and a neurosurgeon, she turned to the neurosurgeon to her left.

"Mr. Siwa, would you like to assist?"

"Absolutely," he declared as he moved in closer.

Once the spinal defect was fully repaired, it was time to close up the uterus. This, too, required the suturing of multiple layers—a more standard procedure than closing the spinal opening, but one that still required intense focus. Claire welcomed the task at hand, for it meant they were that much closer to completing a successful surgery.

There was an air of calmness in the OR as she and Mr. Siwa began stitching up the first uterine layer. It was as if everyone was breathing a collective sigh of relief now that the most critical part of the surgery was now behind them.

Suddenly Dr. McAdams, the cardiologist who had quietly been monitoring Rhianna's heart through echocardiology, called out. "Fetal heart rate is dropping."

Claire jerked her head up as Kiernan asked, "What is it?"

"One-oh-five. Still dropping."

Claire knew that a normal fetal heart rate was one-ten to one-sixty. If it continued to drop steadily, Rhianna would be heading fast to bradycardia. They could lose her.

For a split second, Claire closed her eyes.

"Doctor!" she heard someone exclaim urgently.

Given that the title covered half of the OR team, she couldn't be sure who it was directed to, but it didn't matter at this point. Rhianna's life—perhaps even Jan's—was in her hands now.

"We're in bradycardia," the cardiologist announced, his booming voice momentarily drowning out all the mechanical beeps and hurried voices in the room.

Claire swung her head from the direction of the cardiologist's voice to Kiernan. They locked eyes for a fraction of a second, and in that moment time stood still for Claire. There was no sound, no movement—no anything.

And then…it all came crashing back.

"Increase maternal oxygen," Claire instructed,

knowing that doing so would improve Rhianna's oxygen levels as well.

As Sebastian adjusted Jan's oxygen levels, Kiernan asked, "What's her blood pressure?"

"One-ten over eighty," replied the nurse monitoring vital signs.

If the pressure was low, they could increase it through IV fluids and ephedrine, which in turn would improve blood flow to Rhianna. But it was within normal range.

She shared a look with Kiernan, and knew he was thinking the same thing as her. Aggressive intervention was needed to save Rhianna, and they didn't have a boatload of options.

Though fetal surgery had been inching its way into a viable solution for a growing list of congenital disorders, it was—as Claire's fetal surgery mentor at Boston General, Dr. Eugene Martin, would often say—"Still in its infancy, if you'll pardon the pun."

"Start a fetal IV of point-zero-one milligrams epinephrine," Claire said, shutting off the part of her mind that was one step short of inwardly screaming, *Hurry!*

"An IV?" the closest nurse to her asked.

Rather than be annoyed by the question in the midst of an emergency, Claire replied with a simple, "Yes."

She understood the need for confirmation. To say that she was navigating through uncharted waters was an understatement. Fetal bradycardia was a relatively rare complication during open fetal surgery, but it had been known to happen. Still, there was no definitive protocol in place.

Releasing some of the stitches to pull Rhianna's tiny forearm through, Claire inserted the IV needle and held her breath as Dr. Fleming administered the medication through the IV line. Thirty seconds went by—or was it thirty minutes? Claire knew it was the former, but with Rhianna's life in the balance, it felt like an eternity.

She turned to the cardiologist, who shook his head. "Still dropping. Eighty-seven."

"Atropine?" Kiernan suggested, just as Claire was about to call for it.

She nodded. "I need point-zero-zero-five milligrams atropine."

Dr. Fleming quickly administered the medication. Now all they could do was wait an agonizing minute to see if it worked.

Tick-tick-tick...

"No response!" the cardiologist said, just short of a shout.

Kiernan's ability to remain coolly detached through the most dire of surgical circumstances was being severely tested as the unthinkable began to unfold before him.

They couldn't lose Rhianna. They just couldn't.

It had been his idea to do this surgery here, and Rhianna's death would be on him. Not only would he be responsible for Jan losing her baby, but the loss would destroy Claire—a realization that nearly rendered him immobile. But now was not the time to freeze up. If ever he'd needed to shut off his emotions and focus solely on averting disaster, it was now.

"I'm going to start chest compressions," he said as he leaned over Jan's abdomen.

Across the table, Claire squeezed a hand into the reopened uterus and lifted Rhianna up so that her chest was well into view. But it wasn't enough.

"I'm going to lift her out," Claire said as she pulled Rhianna's head and chest through, leaving the rest of her body inside the womb.

Using his forefinger and middle finger, Kiernan began gently but rapidly compressing the center of Rhianna's chest at a rate of one hundred and twenty compressions per minute. At the sixty-second mark, he swung his head in the direction of Dr. McAdams.

Without needing to be asked, the cardiologist blurted out, "Eighty-five."

Kiernan couldn't see Claire's face beneath the mask, but he knew her grave expression matched his.

"Give another point-zero-one milligrams of epinephrine," she said urgently.

Kiernan halted compressions as Dr. Fleming administered the medication.

"We're still at eighty-five," Dr. McAdams called out twenty seconds later.

"Atropine?" Dr. Fleming asked, a syringe at the ready.

"Yes—point-zero-zero-five milligrams."

Tick-tick-tick...

"Eighty!" came the cardiologist's one-word update.

"Start compressions again," Claire said to Kiernan.

He quickly complied, with a laser-sharp focus, as he strived to deliver the precise amount of pressure.

"Heart rate is increasing. Ninety-eight," said the cardiologist.

Another ten compressions.

"One-twenty."

Kiernan's hand froze as he waited, desperately hoping that Rhianna's heart rate would stabilize.

"One-thirty-seven." Another ten seconds passed. "Heart rate is holding."

"Let's give it another minute to be sure before we start reclosing the uterus," Claire said, her voice a steady beacon in the quiet chaos of the operating theater.

Turning back to Kiernan, she gave a brief nod, as if to say, *I think we got through it.*

Forty-five minutes later Jan was wheeled out into Recovery, all of her vital signs, and Rhianna's, holding steady.

Kiernan watched as Claire walked over to the far side of the room, leaning up against the wall and removing her mask to take a deep and unfiltered breath of air.

"You were amazing," Kiernan said as he walked up beside her.

Claire looked up, her expression exhausted and yet exhilarated at the same time. "So were you. You saved Rhianna's life."

"*We* saved her life."

Claire smiled wearily. "Listen to us. We're debating over who did more to save Rhianna. It was a team effort all the way."

Kiernan's smile was as tired as Claire's, but also as genuine. "You're right. What matters most is that Jan and her baby are both safe and it truly was the best possible outcome."

He paused, wanting so badly to brush back the loose lock of silky chestnut hair that had spilled out of Claire's surgeon's cap. Fighting the urge, he forced himself to briefly look away. But wait… It was officially after the surgery, right? Which meant his self-imposed *don't touch* rule had expired.

He turned back to Claire just as she was pulling off her cap, her hair tumbling perfectly around her shoulders. *Really?* Every lock of hair had just fallen into exactly the right place, with nothing for him to brush aside?

She tilted her head, eyes perplexed. "What's wrong?"

Kiernan mustered up a smile. "Nothing. I was just going to suggest we go and talk to Jan's husband."

"Yes—good idea. I'm sure he'll be relieved… I

can only imagine how worried he must have been this whole time."

And with good reason, Kiernan wanted to say as the earlier emergency played out in quick snippets in his mind.

After sharing the good news with Dave and Jan's two children in the waiting room, Kiernan escorted Claire back into the corridor.

"That is one happy father-to-be," he noted.

Claire smiled. "It feels good, being part of that happiness."

He wanted to probe further, to ask if the successful surgery had shifted anything for her career-wise, but he knew it was way too soon.

Claire bent her neck from side to side, then rubbed her shoulder. "Well, I think I'm going to head back to the cottage and take a nice, long, celebratory hot shower."

Kiernan was *so* tempted to offer to help loofah her back, and pretty much every other square inch of her beautiful, soft skin... But instead he cleared his throat and looked back at her with widened eyes that he did his best to minimize.

"That sounds like a good idea."

"I'll see you tomorrow for our country walkabout. Oh—and please tell Jan's care team to call me if there are any issues. Everything's looking good, and I'm not expecting any complications to crop up, but just in case."

"Will do."

She started down the corridor, turning back briefly to wave and flash an ear-to-ear smile.

"Enjoy your shower!" Kiernan called out, before cringing to himself.

Geez, did I just say that?

As Claire disappeared from view Kiernan had a sinking feeling in the pit of his stomach. He would see her again—for the time being. But the day was coming fast when that would no longer be the case.

And the feeling that was welling up inside him… the almost desperate realization that one day soon she'd be out of his life… Where was it coming from?

Because it wasn't anything he had ever felt for a woman before.

CHAPTER TEN

CLAIRE GLANCED AT her watch as Kiernan's SUV rolled up to her cottage. It was eleven fifty-nine a.m.

One minute early, she mused to herself as their "country walkabout"—destination still unknown—was about to commence.

The digital screen on her watch flashed as the display shifted to twelve p.m.

Or not.

So now she could add "punctual" to the list of Kiernan's attributes, which so far included "talented, brilliant, handsome, athletic, humorous and caring" among others. Although…could someone who was truly caring opt to live a life with no family of his own?

She frowned at her own line of thinking. It was a silly and unfair question. Some people opted to be married to their job, and in Kiernan's case the job entailed helping others—and often saving lives. So wasn't that a type of extended family? Kind of? Sort of?

"Hi."

Claire closed the cottage door behind her and greeted Kiernan. Standing by the SUV passenger door, a casual smile on his face, he looked both unassuming and ruggedly smoldering at the same time.

Claire's next breath caught in her throat.

Whew! Is it getting hot out here?

"What do you know?" Kiernan said, breaking into a smile. "We're twinning."

Claire's eyes had been so laser-focused on Kiernan that she hadn't seen the forest for the trees. Or, more precisely, she hadn't actually noticed what he was wearing. A closer inspection, and she began to laugh.

"You're right," she said as she took note of his jeans, white T-shirt, navy windbreaker and hiking shoes—all of which matched her own attire. "Great minds think alike."

"And dress alike, too," he said with a wink as he held the passenger door open for her.

As their drive got underway, Claire asked the question that had been uppermost in her mind. "How is Jan doing?"

"I checked in on her before leaving the hospital today. She's doing quite well, all things considered. She said Dave and the kids had come by to see her in the morning and were heading back for evening visiting hours."

"That's great to hear."

"She asked about you."

Claire did a double-take. "She did?"

Kiernan turned to her briefly before focusing back on the road. "You seem surprised. She's very grateful that you took on this surgery and wants to make sure you know this."

Claire was genuinely touched. "Please tell her I'm so happy to hear she and Rhianna are doing well."

Kiernan cleared his throat, hesitating for a moment before continuing, "You could come by the hospital and tell her yourself—if you're comfortable with that. I'm sure she'd be thrilled to see you."

Claire looked out the passenger window to collect her thoughts. "It's not that I don't want to see Jan. But I don't want to encroach on Dr. Fleming and her team. I'm sure they're all doing a wonderful job with postoperative care. They deserve credit, too."

She wondered if Kiernan could see through her explanation, which was half truthful and half flimsy excuse. The half that was truth was that she was afraid to get further involved in Jan's journey. Everything was headed in the right direction, and that was how she wanted to remember the experience. The more positives she could build on, the more she might be willing to fully step back into that world someday.

"Are you sure that's all it is?" Kiernan turned to her, seemingly holding his breath for several moments. "I know you came here to try to figure out if you can recommit to your career. If the reason you don't want to come by to see Jan is because you're still grappling with that, I can understand. Although I'm not going to lie... Seeing how happy you were after the surgery was successful, I just thought…"

His voice trailed off, but Claire knew where he was headed. "I know. You thought I'd finally got over the hurdle that's been holding me back." She paused. "I wish I could say it was that easy. And maybe it did help being in a different hospital and in a whole other country. There are so many memories back in Boston."

"I'm sorry. I shouldn't pressure you like this." Another short but meaningful sideways glance. "It's just that you're such an amazing doctor, and I know you still have so much to give. But ultimately I just want for you whatever will make you happiest."

"Me, too," Claire said quietly. "And I feel like I'm on the cusp of figuring it all out." She conjured up a smile as he briefly turned to her once more, his kind brown eyes locking onto hers. "I'm working on it, I promise."

Twenty-five minutes later, Kiernan pulled into the Connemara National Park visitors' center. "We're not visiting the center," he said with a wink. "We're hiking on the Diamond Hill Trail. It's one of the most popular hiking spots in the country." As they exited the SUV, he added, "But we'll be veering off the beaten path in pursuit of one of those hidden gems I mentioned earlier."

Claire raised an eyebrow. "A hidden gem? I'm intrigued."

Kiernan grinned, then stepped around the back

of the SUV and lifted up the hatch door. He pulled out two walking sticks, handing one to Claire.

"You can't go for a walkabout in Ireland without a shillelagh. I carved it myself."

Claire's eyes lit up as she ran her hand over the smooth exterior. Some women got excited over expensive jewelry, but not her.

Give me a genuine shillelagh, hand-carved by a dreamboat surgeon, and I'm the richest woman on the planet.

Looking up at Kiernan, she asked, "What are you—some kind of Renaissance man?"

He chuckled. "I've been called worse." Reaching again into the back of the SUV, he pulled out a large olive-green backpack. "I forgot to tell you to save room for lunch."

"I ate an energy bar just before you picked me up, but don't worry. I always work up an appetite when I'm out moving around in fresh air."

A thick lock of dark hair tumbled over Kiernan's left eye as he dipped down slightly to strap the backpack in place. "Good," he replied as he straightened back up with a mischievous twinkle in his eye. "That could come in handy."

Did he mean...?

Claire grinned, their earlier near-kiss front and center in her mind.

Ten minutes later they were on their way down a path that twisted and turned like a slate-gray version of the yellow brick road.

"There aren't many people here," Claire observed as she looked as far ahead as her vision allowed.

She could see several moving specks that she assumed were fellow hikers, but other than that they had the wide-open trail to themselves.

"It's a weekday, and still a bit early in the season," Kiernan said. "I've been here on weekends in late June and the trail entrance is like the starting gate at a horse race."

Claire wrinkled her nose. "Nothing against other humans, but I'd rather hike alone. Present company the exception, of course."

Kiernan smirked at her comment, adding, "I second that."

Another thing they had in common, Claire thought as they fell into an easy stride. Though the early-spring air held a faint chill, the afternoon sun was warm on her cheeks. She took a deep breath and soaked in her surroundings, and the panoramic view of gently sloping moors dotted with boulders and low mountains in the distance covered in mist.

Thump, step, thump, step, thump, step....

"You know, I've never actually used a walking stick before, but I have to say this really does help you get into a rhythm."

"And you thought Guinness was Ireland's most coveted contribution to the masses."

Claire chuckled. "You do have a way with words." Anticipating his reply, she beat him to the punch. "I know—it's the Gift of the Blarney."

Amused, Kiernan glanced sideways at her.

"Matching outfits and now you're reading my mind. Should I be worried?"

Claire wanted to joke back, except his observation had hit a little too close to the mark. More likely the question was, should *she* be worried that she was enjoying his company so much?

The rapport that she shared with Kiernan was so natural, and so real, that it prompted her to rethink her entire relationship with Mark. Yes, he had turned into someone she no longer recognized, and it still haunted her knowing he had managed to pull the wool over her eyes for so long, shattering her trust in the process. But even before that, back when she'd *thought* they had something good together, it had still never been at this level, nor as easy and effortless.

But soon you'll be out of each other's lives.

The inevitable reminder left a pang in Claire's side, and it was one that she needed to heed. Her mind raced for a way to quickly change the subject, and there was one that was literally in hand.

"What kind of wood is this?" she asked as she held up her shillelagh.

"Blackthorn."

"Sounds prickly."

"It is. The shoots have thorns that can grow up to four inches. Let's just say I practically had to wear an iron hazmat suit when I cut off the branches."

"You definitely are a study in contradictions."

Kiernan glanced at her curiously. "How's that?"

She shrugged. "I haven't known many surgeons who play rugby and carve walking sticks."

"There must be an American equivalent. Surgeons who play tag football and carve pumpkins?"

Claire snickered. "I suppose."

Fifteen minutes later, Kiernan slowed down and pointed to the left. "Here's where we branch off the main path."

Claire cupped her eyes and looked out onto the western landscape. There was nothing obvious that set it apart from the terrain ahead if they stayed on the official trail, but Claire trusted that Kiernan had his reasons for the diversion. Plus, it added to the spirit of adventure, and that could only be a good thing.

They continued on, this time with no words, each taking in the breathtaking scenery as they navigated the slightly uneven terrain.

Another ten minutes passed before Claire broke the silence. "I can see why you choose to live out here in the country, rather than in the city."

Kiernan turned to her. "What about you? I know you work in Boston, but is that where you live as well?"

"I live in Wayland, which is a suburb just west of Boston. It's pretty built up, but there are some pockets of nature here and there."

"That's good."

The conversation dropped off as they continued their climb, and Claire wondered if it was in part due to the subject matter.

You live here. I live there.

Strip away the niceties, and that was what was left. A reminder that they came from two different worlds. And soon she would be returning to hers.

She winced as this reality sank in. The fact that she'd resume her life in Boston after a month in Ireland had always been a given. But then, she hadn't planned on meeting someone like Kiernan.

She turned to him, wondering if he could possibly know that being in his presence made her feel more blissfully alive…and far less tethered to the hurtful past…than she had in a very long time. His eyes were cast downward as he scanned the uneven ground for safe footing, but when he suddenly looked over at her, she blurted out a question to segue from her own thoughts.

"So, you mentioned you grew up in Ballyledge. Did your dad work at West Mercy as well?"

"No, he worked at St. Joseph's Hospital in Dublin."

"That sounds like quite a commute."

"He had an apartment in Dublin."

"Oh…" Claire grimaced, thinking that something in this equation wasn't adding up.

Kiernan turned to her in mid-stride. "You're wondering if he was living a double life of sorts."

"I am?"

Of course she was—not that it felt appropriate to admit as much.

"Well, that's what I'd be wondering if someone told me their father had his own apartment two hundred kilometers away. Which wouldn't necessarily raise red flags if he was divorced from my mother, but that wasn't the case."

"She didn't mind the arrangement?"

"I don't think she felt like she had a say in the matter."

Claire balked, failing to hide her displeasure at this latest revelation. "Sorry," she said quietly.

"Don't be. My mother deserved better, for sure. As to whether my father had a secret second family in Dublin—I honestly don't think so. At least I hope not, given that he couldn't live up to his responsibilities as a husband and father with his first family. And the crazy part—or maybe not so crazy—was that his father, my grandfather, was cut from the same cloth."

"He was a surgeon, too?"

"Yup. And an absentee husband and father."

Claire slowed to a stop.

It was only when Kiernan was several steps ahead of her that he realized she was no longer by his side. He swiveled around, an expression of slight alarm on his face. "Are you okay?"

"You can break the cycle, you know."

Confusion replaced alarm. "What?"

Claire bit her lower lip.

It's now or never. Say what you need to say.

A few moments passed as she tried to muster up some courage. Scanning the immediate vicinity, her gaze landed on a large, flattish boulder that seemed almost too perfect a find. Perhaps the universe was conspiring with her.

"Come sit with me for a minute," she said to Kiernan, before nodding toward the boulder.

Before he could reply, Claire took a seat, leaving plenty of room for Kiernan to join her. He slowly sat down beside her, leaving only the hint of a gap between them. She could feel the warmth of his body and smell his spicy aftershave. Not exactly helpful as she tried to concentrate on the point she needed to make.

"Thanks," she said. "I needed a break."

"No, you didn't," Kiernan said, squinting as he sized her up with the sun in his eyes. "In fact, I'm beginning to think you might be a secret marathoner. I'm feeling slightly winded climbing this hill, and your respiratory rate is on a par with a sloth's."

"You know, I could take offense at that." Claire laughed nonetheless.

Kiernan grinned. "Don't. I meant it in the best possible way."

A cloud must have covered part of the sun, because suddenly his face was partially shaded. No longer squinting, his eyes now displayed the hint of a twinkle.

"So, you were saying that I could break the cycle. Meaning, I suppose, that I can be the first surgeon in my family to not be a selfish jerk."

Claire was taken aback by his blunt assessment, both figuratively and literally. She pulled her torso forward so that she was once again sitting fully upright. "That's not what I meant at all."

"And, for the record, it's only selfish if a man chooses to have a family knowing that he can't give them what they deserve."

Claire widened her eyes at Kiernan's attempted clarification. He was digging his heels in, that was for sure.

"All I meant was, just because both your father and grandfather took the same approach to career versus family, you might think you can't possibly do things differently. But you can."

Kiernan studied Claire closely, his eyes burning into hers. "The old nature versus nurture argument. Is it something genetic that made them both brilliant surgeons but lousy husbands and fathers? Or did my father learn it from his dad, who learned it from who knows who?" He momentarily looked up at the sky in thought. "Come to think of it, my great-great-grandfather was a doctor, too, although I can't vouch for his parenting skills—or lack thereof."

"I just don't want to see you sell yourself short, that's all. Or go through life settling for less than you can have."

Kiernan nodded, and was silent for several moments. Then, "So you always knew you wanted a family, despite what I would imagine is a fairly grueling career as an ob-gyn at a major hospital like Boston General?"

Claire inwardly winced.

Breathe. You prodded him to get this opening. Now make the most of it.

"Yes and no. As in yes, I knew I wanted a family, but no, I wasn't certain I could be fully engaged in my career and also be there for a child in the way that I'd want to be."

As Kiernan pursed his lips together, Claire could almost see the wheels turning in his mind.

"So what made you decide that you could, in fact, do both?"

"When you work with mothers and babies, you see a lot of miracles. And to be a part of making those miracles happen is just the best feeling in the world. But there were times when I'd watch one of these happy endings play out in front of my eyes and it would suddenly dawn on me… Was it right to deny myself that same kind of happiness in order to help bring it to others? You can't go into medicine at a high level, like we have, and not sacrifice something for your career. But was it too great a sacrifice? That's the question I kept asking myself. And ultimately I decided that it was."

"Did you start to approach your career differently once you'd made that decision?"

"I suppose I did—but not in any way that would negatively impact my patients." A slight smile formed on Claire's lips. "Basically, I learned to say no."

Kiernan raised a curious eyebrow. "Oh?"

"No, I'm not going to be regularly putting in twelve-plus-hour days. No, I'm not going to be answering emails at midnight. No, I'm not going to spend *all* my free time at medical conferences or adding more credentials after my name—unless it's something I specifically need to better treat my patients."

She paused for a moment of self-reflection.

"Maybe I couldn't have taken that stance as a resident. But once I paid my dues, I had to rethink my boundaries. And, truth be told, I'm a better doctor for it."

Kiernan half smiled. "Happy doctor, happy patient?"

Claire grinned. "Exactly."

Kiernan looked out onto the rocky yet still lush landscape, his eyes seemingly fixated on a distant object. Was he weighing her take on balancing career and family? She hoped he was at least considering that there were other possibilities besides the one he was so rigidly holding on to.

"I'm glad you shared this," he said quietly. "And I know you'll have another child when the time is right. You have so much love to give."

"Be sure to mention that to the future father—whoever he may be. I want to make sure I don't unknowingly blow him off before things have a chance to get off the ground."

Claire briefly smirked at her own comment, but it was clear that Kiernan didn't share her amusement. His forehead was creased, his eyes pained.

Perhaps he knew her seeming irreverence was an attempt to mask her discomfort.

"That was a stupid thing to say," she said quietly. She waited for his reply, but none was forthcoming. "Well, should we get back on the trail?" she asked, after more silence ensued.

"There's no trail where we're headed, remember?" Kiernan replied with a slight chuckle.

But he had to know that she was deliberately diverting the conversation, and Claire was glad that he knowingly went along with it. As he turned to check his backpack, his shoulder brushed against hers. It felt as strong and as solid as Claire had imagined it would—courtesy, no doubt, of rough-and-tumble rugby rather than the lifting of a scalpel.

"Come on," Kiernan said as he rose from the boulder. "Let's cover some more ground and then we can break for lunch. I have the perfect spot in mind."

No more proselytizing, Claire silently instructed herself.

Today was supposed to be a carefree, take-your-temporary-colleague-on-a-tour day. Couldn't she just go with the flow and enjoy herself?

As she clasped Kiernan's outstretched hand and hopped off the boulder, she had her answer. His grip, firm yet gentle—oxymoron though that might be—was enough to send a jolt through the length of her body. She couldn't be sure what the future held. Not for Kiernan, nor for herself. But she unequivocally knew that in this moment there was no one she would rather be with than the man standing before her now.

You can break the cycle.

Kiernan played the words over again and again in his head, grateful that in a world where it seemed every thought and action were documented in some form of social media, his brain was still a safe haven for every idea and emotion that passed through.

Was he in fact merely repeating what he *assumed* to be true? That dedicated surgeons couldn't successfully split their focus between their career and a family?

Looking back, he couldn't recall a time when he had ever felt differently. And the pushback that had inevitably cropped up in past romantic relationships, the "but of course you can do both" refrains? They had gone in one ear and out the other, accompanied in short order with his own refrain:

I don't think this relationship is going to work.

Done. End of story.

Of course he was exaggerating to himself to think that he had been able to cut all ties so easily. He was human, after all, and he did have a heart—though he sometimes kept that fact well hidden. But what *was* entirely accurate was that no one had ever made him truly question his beliefs. That was until now.

He turned to look at Claire as they forged ahead.

With her eyes intently focused on the uneven grassy terrain beneath their feet, she was oblivious to his stare. Which was good. The last thing he wanted to do was unnerve her with his secret rapt attention.

In the late midday sun, Claire's chestnut hair took on redder tones, and her fair complexion was virtually translucent. She possessed a physical beauty that, quite literally, took his breath away. But it was so much more than that. To know everything she had been through, and see her willingness to potentially invite more personal pain through selflessly taking on Jan's surgery…now *that* was a thing of beauty.

"Is something wrong?" Claire asked, startling Kiernan and dismantling his thoughts.

"No—why do you ask?"

She smiled a bit nervously. "You're looking at me like I have two heads."

Kiernan squashed a wide-eyed grimace before it could fully take hold. "Sorry about that. I was… um…just thinking about something and I guess I was staring without realizing it."

Lame, lame, lame, he silently scolded himself.

"I do the same thing," she said casually, prompting an equally silent *phew*.

"The spot I had in mind for a lunch break is just over that next hill," he said, eager to change the subject.

"Sounds good."

"Your shillelagh holding up okay?"

Claire smiled. "It sure is. In fact, I don't think I'll ever hike again without one."

"Awesome. And, by the way, if you look down near the bottom, you'll see a little something that I carved into the wood for you."

Claire halted and lifted up the bottom of the stick. She twisted it clockwise until the small carved lettering came into view. "'To Claire,'" she read aloud. "'One step at a time. Kiernan.'" She turned to him, momentarily speechless. "Thank you," she said finally, her voice both soft and sincere. "Words to live by, for sure."

Kiernan pursed his lips together and nodded. "You're very welcome."

He had added the message earlier in the morning, before picking up Claire, an idea that had only partially been on a whim. The desire to leave something with Claire that she could always remember him by had been percolating in his mind for several days. That it would be a message on a walking stick had been a last-minute choice, but it had felt so right when it came to him that he hadn't second-guessed the decision.

"Whew!" Claire declared fifteen minutes later, when they had nearly finished descending the final hill before lunch. She removed her windbreaker and tied it around her waist. "The sun is really starting to throw some heat."

"I know," Kiernan agreed. "It feels good."

He scanned the area once they were back on level ground, looking for familiar landmarks. It didn't take long to spot them. A heavy concentration of large boulders lining another hill about one hundred meters ahead and to the left, thick brush to the right, and a narrow grassy passageway in between.

He pointed to a stone ledge at the start of the rocky hill. "We can lunch there."

It was a short climb to the naturally formed perch, and he wasted no time sliding the backpack off his shoulders.

"Heavy?" Claire asked.

"Heavy enough," he replied with a rueful smile, stretching his neck to both sides to work out some of the kinks.

"Let me guess… Deep-dish, three-cheese lasagna?" Claire quipped as he unzipped the backpack.

Kiernan chuckled. "Even better. I decided to ditch my usual lunch of greasy sausage and chips for something healthier."

Claire grimaced. "Sausage and chips? Seriously? That's probably what brought your carotid endarterectomy patient into the OR today."

"Be quiet, you."

Claire smirked. "Just saying. And by the way— how did the surgery go?"

"It was fairly routine and by the book. He'll be back home tomorrow, and hopefully he will start following some of the healthy eating guidelines that one of our dieticians will be going over with him."

"You mean the ones you don't follow yourself?"

Kiernan feigned insult—not easy to do, given

that he was actually quite amused. "I don't think I've seen this feisty side to you before."

"That's what happens when I'm hungry. I get a little obnoxious."

"Remind me to carry snacks around at all times," Kiernan quipped as he extracted two brown bags out of the backpack. "One for me and one for you. Chickpea spread sandwiches with baked—not fried—crisps. And don't blame me if the sandwich tastes like…"

"Chickpeas?" Claire offered teasingly.

"I was going to say chalk."

"I love chickpeas. Good choice. And definitely a step above cucumbers."

Kiernan chuckled as he handed her a bottle of seltzer water and then leaned back, with a boulder behind him doubling as a backrest. He scanned the thicket across the way, looking for any sign that a certain four-legged dweller was still in the area. Suddenly, a swatch of white flashed within the twisted tangles of brown vegetation.

Kiernan gently grabbed Claire's forearm and pointed with his other hand. "There. Do you see her?"

Claire strained to view the area, then gasped. "Yes…yes, I see her! She's beautiful!" She turned to Kiernan, eyes wide with wonder. "I didn't realize there were white foxes in Ireland."

"There aren't. Well, not as a species. She's albino. I first spotted her two springs ago and I thought the same thing, too. White foxes in Ireland? But I did a little research and, though it's extremely rare, there is such a thing as an albino red fox."

As Claire leaned in slightly and squinted, Kiernan quietly pulled a pair of binoculars from the backpack. "I brought them just in case."

Claire peered into them for several moments. "I see two babies with her. Not white."

She handed the binoculars to Kiernan, and he confirmed her observation.

"She has a burrow somewhere in the thicket. To be honest, when I first spotted her two years ago, I never thought I'd see her the following year."

"You mean because she can't blend into her surroundings?"

"Exactly. She's even more vulnerable to predators than a normal fox. But since that first time I've had five sightings in total, the last one being in November."

"Her ears just pricked up," Claire said as she peered through the binoculars. "Oh—she's looking right at me."

"I'd say she can smell the chickpea sandwich, but I'm sure she'd prefer chips and sausages."

Claire smiled at the comment. "She's turning around now. There she goes—back with her babies into the brush."

"Her den's in there and she's being a protective mum."

Claire nodded and rested the binoculars beside her. "Not a bad thing."

"Nope. Safety first."

Claire looked earnestly into his eyes, and this time he held her gaze. "Thank you for bringing me here. You're right—it's a hidden gem."

"I'm glad you think so."

Claire wasn't looking away, and neither was he. His eyes fell to her pillowy lips...those same luscious lips he had come so close to kissing under a moonlit sky as ocean breezes danced around them. He had thought *that* had been the perfect, albeit missed, moment. But being this close to Claire... seeing the desire in her eyes that matched his own...feeling a connection to her that was deeper than he had ever felt for a woman...*this* was the perfect moment. And he was going to make it last.

Every. Spine-tingling. Second.

As he slowly moved in closer, she met him halfway. Their lips touched, and he felt as though he had been waiting for this kiss his whole life. Perhaps he had. Which was why he had no intention of rushing through it. He savored every exquisite sensation: the sweet softness of her lips, the silky luster of her hair as he ran his fingers through it, the warmth of her breath on his cheek as they slowly pulled back, only to reengage...

It was deeper and longer and more satiating than he had imagined their kiss could be. And he had been imagining it from almost the first time he had laid eyes on Claire.

Moments—no, make that minutes...*many* minutes later, they reluctantly parted lips and leaned back on the rock.

"Wow," Claire said, looking slightly dazed but altogether pleased.

"I second that," Kiernan said.

And third and fourth...

"Are you sure you weren't just trying to get me to work up an appetite for that chickpea sandwich?"

Kiernan chuckled. "Am I that transparent?"

Claire leaned over and grabbed one of the sandwiches, then delicately took a bite as Kiernan watched.

"Well?" he asked.

She shrugged her shoulders. "Eh…maybe I'm just not hungry right now."

An impish grin gave away her ruse, and he placed a hand just above her knee as he pulled himself closer again. "Then you give me no choice but to work more on that appetite."

"If you insist."

As he caressed her back and pulled her close, Kiernan replied, "I most certainly do."

It was still light outside but heading toward dusk as Kiernan pulled up to Claire's cottage. She turned to him while remaining seated. "Thanks. I had a great time. Make that a *really* great time."

"Me, too."

"And I love the shillelagh. I might need to book its own seat on the flight home, but it's well worth it."

Though Kiernan grinned at her joke, this reminder of the transient nature of her stay was anything but amusing.

Seeing her hand on the door handle, he quickly changed the subject. "Despite my insistence that I could take time off during the week, it's not looking like I can break away from the hospital for another outing before the weekend. One of my general surgeons broke his ankle stepping in a rabbit hole."

"Don't tell me—he was playing golf?"

Kiernan rolled his eyes. "He was. And now I have to fill in for some of his surgeries. But I'm free this Saturday, if you're up for another adventure. No chickpea sandwiches, I promise."

"Sounds like a plan." She stepped out of the SUV and turned back. "Call or text me about when you plan to come by, and I'll see you then."

"Wait—I think you're forgetting something."

Her quizzical expression quickly eased into a smile. Leaning back into the car, she readily kissed him before finally pulling away to exit the vehicle once more.

As Kiernan watched her walk to the cottage he briefly closed his eyes. He had never been one to jump on the *life can be so unfair* bandwagon, but it sure as heck felt like the universe was conspiring against him. How else to explain that he had met a woman who took his breath away on every level, but soon she'd be out of his life for good?

He opened his eyes just in time to see Claire wave to him before disappearing into the cottage. With a deep sigh, he put the SUV in "drive." It was equipped with a GPS that had never led him astray. If only he had the equivalent of such a device for his heart. Because that earlier directive of "just enjoy the moment while she's here?" It no longer felt like a viable destination.

CHAPTER ELEVEN

CLAIRE STARED OUT the cottage window as she leaned over the back of the couch, her phone plastered against her ear. Only two rings into the call, her sister promptly answered.

"Claire—it's so good to hear from you! How's it going over there? Meet any hunky Irishmen?"

Claire managed to crack a smile as she shook her head. "No comment."

Her sister was quick to reply. "Whoa—that means yes!"

Claire turned back from the window, her thoughts very much on a particular hunky Irishman. If there were others in existence she didn't know, and quite frankly didn't care.

"Well?" Grace asked, disrupting Claire's *very* enjoyable thoughts.

Grace was not only her sister, but also her best friend. At home, they talked on the phone, often with video, at least four or five times a week. But before coming to Ireland, Claire had made a pledge to herself that she would limit her calls with Grace to no more than a few in total. She had come here to break free of the past and to contemplate her future—and doing so meant uncoupling from reminders of home. Even those reminders that she cared about. Their only previous call had been on the day she'd landed, to say that she had arrived safely. Which meant there was a whole lot of ground to cover.

Taking a deep breath, Claire fully dove in and filled Grace in on Margaret and Kiernan, and Jan and Kiernan…and Kiernan and Kiernan and Kiernan.

"Oh, my gosh," Grace said breathlessly. "Here I was joking around, but you really *did* meet a hunky Irishman. And another doctor, no less."

"Surgeon," Claire corrected.

"There's a difference?"

Claire smiled ruefully. "According to most surgeons, yes."

"I have so many questions that I don't even know where to begin. Let me start with the obvious one."

"Okay, I'll bite. What's the obvious question?"

"Is he a good kisser?"

Claire laughed while simultaneously feeling her cheeks grow hot. "No."

"Really?"

"He's better than good. But that's all I'm going to tell you."

"Oh, come on, now! I've been married for about a gazillion years—I need some vicarious thrills."

Claire snickered softly, but she was too caught up in her thoughts to answer. Grace's question had sent her right back to that moment when Kiernan had looked deeply into her eyes, pulled her close, and kissed her in a way that had made every previous kiss in her life a pale second at best. Or was it more like a pale tenth? Um…a pale *hundredth*?

"Claire?"

"Huh?"

"I asked you if you thought it was possible that things with Kiernan could develop into something more?"

Claire's smile quickly evaporated. Harsh reality had a way of making smiles doing that. "I don't see how, given that we live in different countries. And I told you he doesn't want to have kids."

"Yeah, that's a deal-breaker, for sure. Although maybe you could change his mind."

"Grace, you know what four words have led to the most disappointment in relationships since the beginning of time? *I can change him.* Or, for that matter, *I can change her.*"

Grace sighed. "I know… I know. It's just that when you talk about him I can hear in your voice how happy you are. And I don't think I've heard that in a very long time."

Claire stared at the floor as she contemplated her sister's observation. It was true that Kiernan had a way of making her feel more alive, and it was a feeling that grew every time she was with him. But that didn't mean they could possibly have a future together. Not when the insurmountable obstacles of living in two different countries, with opposing views on having children, were stacked against them.

"Well, I'm actually on my way to see the man of the hour."

"Kiernan?"

Claire tempered a roll of her eyes with a grin. "No, a leprechaun."

"Ha-ha. Well, good for you. And Claire…?"

After a few moments of silence, Claire spoke. "Were you going to ask me something?"

"I was just wondering if you've made any headway on your decision about your career."

Claire sighed. "Headway, yes. But any definitive game plan of what to do next…not exactly. I came here expecting some quiet time alone to contemplate things. But it's been a crazy whirlwind from the start."

"What about the breech delivery and the fetal surgery, though? You must have felt good about helping those mothers and their babies."

"Of course! I don't think that part of the job ever changes. But it's not always a happy ending like that." She paused. "Maybe I just need to start fresh somewhere else."

"You mean leave Boston General? You love that hospital!"

"I know. I have great colleagues, and I've made some really good friends over the years. But it's hard to separate that from some of the bad feelings I get when I think about the hospital. There are just so many memories there."

Claire knew she didn't have to point out to her sister exactly what she meant. After graduating medical school, both she and Mark had completed their residency at Boston General, with Mark then moving on to private practice. But it still held three years of memories of one of the most exciting times of her life as she'd fully realized her dream of becoming an ob-gyn.

And then, four years later…in Room 471 on the fourth floor in the obstetrics wing…she'd said goodbye to Ariana.

"Well, if you do decide to move on from Boston General, you'll have no problem landing somewhere else, that's for sure," said Grace. "In fact, they'll be lining up to sign you on."

Claire pulled her lips into a tight smile. "Thanks, Sis. But I'm a long way from making such a big decision. One step at a time, I guess."

Her own words momentarily startled her. Whether consciously or not, she had just repeated the message on her walking stick. As if on cue, she heard Kiernan's SUV roll to a stop outside the cottage.

After promising Grace they'd talk again soon, Claire closed the cottage door behind her, then turned to greet Kiernan as he stood by the passenger door. But instead of saying hi, the only word that came out of her mouth was a loud gasp. It was quickly followed by a blink of her eyes—just to make sure they weren't playing tricks on her.

"That is *not* a kilt you're wearing."

Had he read her mind the other night at his place? Kiernan peered down at the green and black plaid tartan skirt, then back up at Claire. "Huh. I could have sworn I put trousers on this morning."

Claire's laughter bordered on a giggle.

"Do you like it?" Kiernan asked as he jokingly twirled around, his rugged body the equivalent of a bull pirouetting in a china shop.

It was a spectacle that promoted even more laughter from Claire.

"I do," she conceded, though she couldn't be sure if she was complimenting the kilt or the black-socked muscular calves that were fully on display. "So, is there a reason for this catchy ensemble?"

"As a matter of fact, there is." He opened the passenger door. "Step inside, lass, and you'll find out soon enough."

Twenty minutes later, the SUV turned off the main road, slowly passed through an open wrought-iron gate, then continued up a narrow paved path. At the top of a hill, a one-tower castle loomed over the lavish landscape.

Claire strained her neck to get a better view from the passenger seat. "What castle is this?"

"Rockminster Castle. Built in 1547 by my great-great-great-great-grandfather on my mother's side. Wait—did I say five greats, or four?"

"I wasn't counting, but I think four."

"Should be five." He turned to Claire, a half-smile on his face. "It was a long time ago."

"Your family has a *castle*? Any other secrets I should know about?"

Kiernan chuckled. "Don't get too excited. It's

a small castle. Kind of the equivalent of a studio apartment in the sixteenth century."

"It looks way bigger than a studio apartment," Claire observed as they drew closer to the structure. "Is it open to the public?"

"Not in any official capacity. My uncle, who lives in town, takes care of the upkeep. He'll rent it out for the occasional photo shoot or tea party on the grounds. That sort of thing… There's some interesting history in the walls of this castle, too."

As they exited the SUV, Claire scanned the post-card-worthy grounds with awe. "So, let's hear about some of that interesting history. Ours doesn't go back nearly as far in America."

Kiernan extracted a key from his pocket and unlocked the deadbolt on the large wooden door at the castle entrance. The air was chilled and musty as they made their way inside.

"Better yet, I'll take you right to the scene where it all happened."

As Claire followed Kiernan, she couldn't imagine a sexier history guide. At the top of a short flight of stairs they entered a small room with a wooden bed against one wall, and a dresser with a wash pan on the other side. A single window with metal bars looked out onto the front grounds. It was hard not to feel claustrophobic in such cramped surroundings, although Claire wondered if more was at play.

Kiernan, on the other hand, seemed unfazed as he began to fill her in on some of the castle's secrets. "Legend has it that at the turn of the seventeenth century, during the Nine Years War with England, the daughter of one of my ancestors fell in love with a British soldier."

"Uh-oh…"

Kiernan grimaced. "Exactly. When her father found out, he had her locked up in this very room, fully intending to keep her here until the war ended and the soldier departed. Or died in battle, I suppose—whichever came first."

Whether real or imaginary, Claire felt a sudden breeze rustle past her, and she wrapped her arms close to her chest in a protective stance.

"Am I scaring you?" Kiernan asked, stepping closer until there was little space between them. "I don't mean to."

"More like I'm scaring myself." She forced a brave smile, but the goosebumps on her arms remained. "So what happened?"

"Well, the daughter—her name was Bronagh—didn't take too well to being locked away. One night, when a castle guard was shoving a plate of food under the door, she asked if she could open the door to speak to him. Of course he said no, but she must have said something to charm him into complying, because he did open the door."

Wide-eyed, Claire blurted out, "And…?"

"She pushed past the guard and ran upstairs onto the watchtower, where she jumped to her death."

Claire flinched, her breath momentarily caught

in her throat. "I think I now have goosebumps on top of my goosebumps."

"You might be feeling the presence of her ghost."

Claire bared her teeth. "Okay, now you're just messing with me."

Kiernan chuckled. "No, it's the truth. Over the years there's been a number of sightings of a young woman in a white frock, gazing out of this window." He pointed just behind Claire. "She stares back…then evaporates into thin air."

"Have you ever seen her?"

"No, but my mum saw her when she was a kid. It scared her so much she's rarely been back here. And my uncle has, on at least half a dozen occasions—including up on the tower where she jumped from. It's up the stairs outside this room. One of the previous groundskeepers saw her there, too."

"Can we go up the tower?" Claire asked, hoping Kiernan would reply quickly, before she lost her nerve.

Kiernan raised an eyebrow. "Are you sure you want to?"

"Are you calling me a scaredy cat?"

Kiernan grinned. "Nope, not me." He nodded to the door.

With Kiernan just behind her, Claire made her way up the narrow stone stairs, which coiled upwards in a clockwise fashion like a tightly wound snake.

"I can see why they didn't need elliptical machines back then," Claire said as she felt the lactic acid building up in her leg muscles with each additional step. "They got a workout just from getting from point A to point B in the castle."

"True," Kiernan replied, though Claire was quite certain *his* legs were finding the laborious climb a breeze.

Finally, a ray of sun broke through the darkness and illuminated the stairs just above her. "I think we're almost there."

A few more steps, and they were at the top of the watchtower. Unlike the small, bar-covered window in the previous room, the tower's windows were much larger and free of any hindrance. It made sense, though morbidly so, that Bronagh had chosen this spot to cast herself to the ground.

Kiernan walked up beside Claire, and together they looked out onto the sun-drenched grounds. "It almost looks too idyllic, considering what happened here," she said quietly.

"I know. Although I've been here on overcast days and you really do feel a different energy." Still staring straight ahead, he said, "And by the way... the name Bronagh means sorrow."

"Wow," Claire said softly. "It's like the plot for a tragic romance—except it really happened. I wonder why she felt she had to go to that extreme. The war wasn't going to last forever, so she had to know that someday she'd be free again."

"I don't know..." Kiernan's gaze remained fixed on the horizon. "I guess people do crazy things for love."

He slowly turned to Claire, his dark eyes melting into her own. She felt her breath catch first, and then her heart.

Stepping in closer, he brushed his fingers along her cheek, then pulled her in until their bodies touched. Without hesitation, he caressed her lips with his own, and time seemed to stand still as the kiss grew deeper and more passionate.

Claire no longer needed to fantasize about the rugby-primed chest beneath his shirt. She could feel each taut muscle as it pushed against her breasts, and the friction of their clothing sent waves of pleasure throughout her body. His lingering kisses along the length of her neck made her weak in the knees, and as Kiernan swept her off her feet and up into his powerful arms all she could do…all she *wanted* to do…was fully melt into the moment.

She closed her eyes and tipped back her head, but as Kiernan determinedly strode back to the staircase, like a man on a mission, she reluctantly popped one eye back open.

"Kiernan," she said breathlessly. "You can't carry me down these crazy stairs."

He playfully brushed his lips against her bottom lip. "Aye, I can. Leave it to me, lass."

Claire wasn't sure whether to laugh at his comment, brace herself for a fall, or kiss him passionately for good luck. So she did all three.

With his body of a bull that had somehow merged with the gracefulness of a gazelle, Kiernan descended the twisting staircase in record time. Entering the small room from where they had started their climb, he gently placed Claire on the bed, but there was a fire in his eyes that she knew was about to engulf them both.

Clothing came off…slowly at first, then at a feverish pitch. And as the timeworn wooden bed creaked Claire wondered if it might snap in half.

Go ahead. Break.

It was easy not to have a care in the world when every nerve-ending quivered with desire…

Kiernan was every bit the incredible lover she had imagined he'd be. And, yes, she had been imagining it a *lot* leading up to this moment. He was attentive, generous, and fully attuned to her on a level that seemed to go far beyond the physical. Every kiss, every whisper, every touch seemed solely designed to bring her pleasure, and she fully responded in kind.

As their lovemaking climaxed into a glorious release she felt something deep inside her shift, as though her healing had reached another apex. Lying quietly together, still wrapped in each other's arms, she could only conclude one thing: the power of love was real.

Later, as they walked in the flower-filled castle grounds, Kiernan reached over and took Claire's hand, their fingers effortlessly interlocking.

"How's Jan doing?" she asked suddenly.

The question caught Kiernan by surprise. Was she trying to deflect the conversation away from the two of them, knowing that the closeness and passion they'd just shared had opened an exhilarating door that would soon be slammed shut? It was a sobering realization that hovered in the back of his own mind, so he couldn't blame her for possibly feeling the same.

"She's doing great," he replied. "In fact, she'll be discharged from the hospital on Tuesday. Her C-section has been scheduled, so it's just a matter of her taking it easy at home for the remainder of the pregnancy."

"Do you think I could see her before she leaves?"

Given Claire's previous reluctance to see Jan again, the question shocked Kiernan—but in the best possible way. Still, knowing that literally jumping for joy in his kilt might not only make her change her mind, but also possibly put the family jewels on full display—*ahem*—he tamped down his outward enthusiasm.

"Of course. Do you want to come by on Monday? Say late morning or early afternoon? That way, I'll be able to pop in for the visit as well." He paused. "Unless you'd rather I didn't?"

Claire grinned. "Of course I want you to be there. And Dr. Fleming, too, if she's available. We were all in this together, and it would be nice to have a little reunion post-surgery."

Hoo, boy! This was progress!

Kiernan discreetly took a deep breath, but there was no hiding his ear-to-ear smile. Not only was he basking in the glow of the intimacy they had just shared, but Claire was taking another step in a career-reengaging direction, and he simply couldn't be happier.

Except....

Kiernan clenched his jaw tight as the other half of this equation revealed itself. Resuming her career meant her returning to Boston General. Which certainly was not a new revelation. But now...no, *especially* now, the thought of Claire leaving Ireland stung. And it stung hard.

Be happy for her, he told himself.

And he was. But that didn't mean he wouldn't miss her for the rest of his life.

Claire and Dr. Fleming were standing by Jan's bedside late on Monday morning when Kiernan entered the room. "I'm sorry I'm late. My last surgery went over a bit," he said hurriedly, his rapid breath screeching to a halt as Claire looked up at him, her green eyes sparkling in the brightly lit room.

"No worries," Dr. Fleming replied. "We've just been chatting with Jan about some of the best online stores for baby girls' clothing. My personal favorite is Tiny Frills. And Claire likes the handmade clothes on Etsy."

Uh-oh. Kiernan felt the muscles in his jaw and neck clench. Of course Dr. Fleming could have no idea how much discomfort this discussion would trigger in Claire. Still, though there was a tightness evident in her smile, Claire seemed to be taking it all in stride.

"Jan is being discharged at ten a.m. tomorrow," Dr. Fleming said. "Then it's home to be with her family until her scheduled C-section at thirty-seven weeks."

"Don't forget I have to take bedrest," Jan said, with an understandable lack of enthusiasm in her voice.

"I know it can seem daunting," Claire replied empathetically. "But I have a feeling the time will fly by."

"And then, before you know it," Dr. Fleming added, "you'll be holding Rhianna in your arms."

Seeing Claire's smile waver for a fleeting second, Kiernan quickly jumped in. "So, have you thought about what your first home-cooked meal will be?"

Claire met his eyes, as if silently thanking him for his not so thinly veiled attempt to change the subject.

"That depends on who's doing the cooking," Jan replied wryly. "I assume it won't be me, so that leaves either Dave or my mum, who's going to be staying with us until Rhianna arrives. Let's just say I know who I *hope* will be playing chef. Don't get me wrong—my husband's good at sharing the chores at home. But he can't properly boil an egg, never mind make an edible meal."

Laughter sounded through the room, and after another ten minutes of easy banter between Jan and the doctors the conversation came to a natural standstill. Finally, Claire filled in the silence.

"Well, Jan, I want to wish you the best with everything. I can now leave Ireland knowing you're in good hands here, with Dr. Fleming and her team."

"Thank you for everything," Jan said earnestly. "And I'd love to send you a picture of Rhianna when she's born."

"That would be wonderful."

Ten minutes later, the visit wound down, and Kiernan and Claire exited the room.

"I'm glad I came by," Claire said, in buoyant spirits at least as far as Kiernan could discern.

"I'm glad you did, too. It was good to get that closure with Jan." He slowed to a halt in the corridor, with Claire following suit. "So, have you thought about how you'll spend your last days here?"

He'd dreaded asking the question, but posed it in the hopes that she might say she had extended her leave.

"I'm not sure. Maybe I'll take a drive up the coast…stay in a bed-and-breakfast for a night."

As a sharp pang of disappointment gripped him, he pivoted to the thought of asking if there might be room for two. But before he could get the words out a door several feet away flew open and a young, cherub-faced nurse with reddened eyes nearly stumbled out of the room.

Kiernan froze in his steps. "What's wrong?" he asked urgently.

The nurse glanced at his nametag, her cheeks now reddening as much as her eyes. "I'm sorry, sir," she said, her voice cracking with emotion.

An older nurse exited the room and gently closed the door behind her.

"Is everything okay, Carol?" Kiernan asked.

She nodded, then placed a comforting hand on the younger nurse's shoulder. "This is Amy's first week…she's fresh out of nursing school," she explained. Turning to her younger colleague, she added, "It never gets easy, seeing something like this, but with time you'll be able to keep your emotions in check."

"What happened?" Claire asked, a hint of dread in her voice.

"A stillborn girl at thirty-four weeks. Dr. O'Conner induced labor nearly forty minutes ago, and both parents have been cradling her ever since. It's quite an emotional scene, as you can imagine." She looked back at the closed door, her forehead creased. "I've told them to take all the time they need. Everyone's different. Sometimes, the parents can't bear to do more than kiss their baby goodbye. Others find it hard to let go."

Kiernan turned to Claire, a sense of disbelief seeping into him that such a positive visit with Jan could be instantly counteracted in the worst possible way.

Instead of meeting his eyes, she stared at the door, and all he could do was hold his breath.

Claire looked at the small square window on the door. Everything told her to remain where she was, that nothing good would come out of peering inside the room. And that was on top of the fact that doing so would be a tremendous invasion of privacy for the grieving parents. But the compulsion building inside her had a mind of its own.

Turning back to Kiernan, she saw the deep concern etched on his face. She smiled and nodded to him as a signal that she was okay, then waited for him to be reluctantly pulled into a conversation with Carol. With his head now turned away from her, Claire discreetly stepped toward the door.

Her glance inside the window could not have lasted more than five seconds. But it was still long enough to imprint the scene on her mind. A couple, presumably husband and wife, clutching each other and sobbing together.

Stepping away from the window, Claire saw Kiernan do a double-take as he glanced back over at her. Had he read the distress on her face? It would have been hard not to at this point. Though she couldn't hear the exact conversation between Kiernan and the two nurses, it was clear from both the inflection of his voice and his fidgety stance that he was trying to wrap things up as quickly as possible.

As the nurses departed, Kiernan was immediately at Claire's side. "Are you okay?"

"Yes. It's just that…" She paused, shaking her head. "I shouldn't have looked in the room."

"I'm sure it brought back painful memories," Kiernan said quietly.

"The husband was holding his wife, and they were both crying. When I lost Ariana, Mark was nowhere to be found. I remember holding her for what seemed like forever, not wanting the doctor to come take her away. And Mark didn't even care."

Kiernan's eyes narrowed, like daggers aimed at an invisible Mark. "Did he know you were in the hospital?"

"I didn't contact him, but one of the nurses did. She really had no right to do that, but she was friends with him. She told me later that he acted all annoyed when she told him that Ariana was about to be stillborn and they were inducing labor. 'Like he couldn't be bothered' was the way she described it to me. She vowed never to talk to him again after that."

Kiernan clenched his jaw. "I'm so sorry you went through this alone. That never should have happened."

Alone. She hadn't really thought much before about how deeply Mark's complete disregard for the loss of their child had affected her, but now she couldn't unsee the connection. Watching that couple grieve together, simultaneously cradling each other and their tiny stillborn daughter—that was how it *should* be. If Mark had been the man she'd initially thought he was—if they'd had a strong marriage and if he had grieved the death of their baby as a loving husband and father should—then perhaps she would have been better equipped to move past the active stage of a trauma that had never fully resolved.

Kiernan wouldn't have left me alone.

That her thoughts had even gone there was almost shocking to Claire. But should it have been, knowing how he had so resolutely stayed by her side through several emotional upheavals?

"Are you okay?" Kiernan asked again, eyeing her intently.

It took several moments for her to nod. "I wasn't expecting this…especially after everything went so well with Jan's visit…but I'm okay. Really."

Less than a month ago she would never have been able to say this. But that had been before Kiernan. Their time together, though counted only in weeks, had impacted her enough for a lifetime, and given her a renewed strength that she'd thought she had lost forever.

But Kiernan appeared less than convinced by her reply.

"Do you want to go to the café, and we can sit and talk for a bit?"

Claire hesitated as she weighed the offer. Though she had just successfully ridden out the surge of emotions prompted by peering into the stillbirth room, something was still niggling at her.

"I think I'm going to head back to the cottage for some duck therapy," she replied finally.

Kiernan smiled, though it didn't completely erase the concern in his eyes. "Can I see you tonight?"

She held his gaze, unable to answer. There was that niggling again, like a tapping against her brain that said, *Yoo-hoo, there's something we need to discuss.*

"I think I'm just going to lay low tonight. But I'll be in touch."

Kiernan pursed his lips together and nodded. He didn't say anything…nor did he have to. The disappointment in his eyes spoke loud and clear.

Later that night, as she stared up at the dark ceiling from her bed, Claire finally acknowledged what had been chipping away at her subconscious since earlier that day. From their initial chance meeting during a high-stakes baby delivery, and culminating in their better-than-she-could-have-imagined tryst in the castle, she had shared an emotional and physical connection with Kiernan unlike any she had ever known.

But today she'd had an unexpected gut-check. And what had it taken for the bubble to finally burst? The fantasy to be replaced with reality? It had been seeing the couple at the hospital who had just lost their baby, and knowing that Kiernan would be the kind of husband and father who'd be there for her if she'd been that grieving mother…

Except for one little thing. He wanted nothing to do with either role. Which was his prerogative, right? Just as it was hers to decide to cut her losses before her heart was further crushed. And that meant telling him goodbye. Not on her last day here. Not at the airport. *Now*.

Claire abruptly turned on her side, as though she could dislodge her distressing thoughts, but they clung to her too tightly. She had known from the get-go that her time in Ireland was temporary and any attachment to Kiernan would be a mistake. But somewhere along the way she'd forgotten—or perhaps willfully ignored—her own warning. It was as if she had started to believe that *this* was her life now. Living in the beautiful Irish country-side, working side by side with Kiernan, her love for him growing every second of every day…

Yes… I said it. My love for him.

Never in a million years had she thought she'd fall so head-over-heels in love during her brief stint in Ireland.

But the heart wants what it wants. Even when it can't have what it wants.

Just shy of a week from now she would again be staring at a dark ceiling—but it would be in the bedroom of her condo just outside of Boston. Somehow, some way, she'd resume her previous life—though it now seemed inevitable that Boston General would not be part of that reunion.

It will all work out, she told herself.

More than once in the past those words had gotten her through the toughest of times. But not so much now. Maybe because the mantra implied that something good could come out of saying goodbye to Kiernan forever. And that, quite frankly, just didn't seem possible.

CHAPTER TWELVE

KIERNAN DUCKED AS a sledgehammer swung precariously close to his head. The fact that it came complete with human fingers and was attached to the gargantuan shoulder of a rugby teammate named Angus did little to alter Kiernan's perception that he was being swiped at with a block of iron on a stick.

"Hey, take it easy," he said as Angus swung out again, this time smacking him hard on the shoulder.

In his boisterous teammate's defense, he realized Angus probably thought he was just giving him a friendly post-game pat—not setting him up for future joint replacement surgery.

"Aye! I'm just a little pumped-up about our win."

Angus grabbed Kiernan in a bear hug, landing a couple of knuckle-knocks on the head for good measure. When he finally broke free, Kiernan laughed at his friend's shenanigans, then joined the rest of the rambunctious group as they tumbled into the main room of Gilroy's Pub.

Almost immediately, he spotted Claire sitting alone at a nearby table.

She waved discreetly, and he wasted no time in heading over.

"This is a pleasant surprise," he said as he pulled out a chair, smiling so deeply that he felt his cheeks would burst.

After their downcast parting of ways at the hospital yesterday, this unexpected reunion was a special treat. Actually, that could be said about *any* time he was in her presence. Which begged the question…was it possible he could find a way to stay in her presence more permanently?

I know… I know…she's leaving soon.

Knowing it wasn't the right time to grapple with such thoughts, Kiernan pushed them aside and focused on the beautiful face in front of him.

Claire smiled, but not with her usual verve. "I wasn't sure if you'd still be playing today, with all the rain we had earlier," she said.

"Are you kidding? Rain means mud, and I swear some of the guys—make that most—prefer a soggy field. It's easier to squash someone's face into the ground."

Claire snickered, but her amusement was short-lived. The smile evaporated and her eyes flashed with angst.

"Are you okay?" he asked gingerly.

"I came here hoping that we could talk."

Coupled with her troubled demeanor, the announcement left Kiernan reeling with dread.

"Yes, of course," he managed to say, as evenly as possible.

She scanned the loud and crowded pub. "It was

raining pretty hard when I got here a half-hour ago. Is it still raining now?"

"No, just a light mist."

"Can we take a walk on the pier?"

"Sure."

As they walked along the pier several minutes later, Claire stopped abruptly and turned to him. "Kiernan, what I'm about to say is not easy for me. As you know, I came here seeking clarity about my career—something that I felt I was never going to find back home, where there are still so many reminders of painful things. But what I didn't expect to happen…" She paused, visibly swallowing twice, as though pushing back emotions. "What I didn't expect was meeting someone I'd develop very strong feelings for."

Only the sound of waves lapping against the pier could be heard as she stared into his eyes. Kiernan wanted to stay silent as he waited for her to resume talking, but he couldn't.

"Claire, I wasn't expecting this either. But is it so bad that we *did* meet each other, and that we *do* have these feelings?"

"For me, yes."

Her reply was like a one-two gut-punch. "I see," was all that he could manage to say.

"I can't be the only one realizing that this can't go anywhere. We don't want the same things, Kiernan. I mean, many things, we do—but not the one thing that I can't compromise on."

"A child," he said quietly.

She nodded. "And I know that I'm getting too far ahead of myself here by even bringing this up. It's not like we're even in a relationship—right?"

Kiernan wasn't sure if this was a genuine or rhetorical question, but he was unable to answer either way.

"And you know what kills me about all of this, what I just can't wrap my head around, is how you insist that you're someone you're not."

What?

Kiernan's head was now officially spinning. He had told Claire why he wouldn't put a child in the position his father had put him in. He'd been honest with her about that.

"I'm not sure what you mean."

"Yesterday, when I looked into that room and saw the husband consoling his wife… Mark wasn't that kind of husband and father. But Kiernan, *you* are."

"But—"

"I know," Claire quickly interjected. "What the heck am I talking about, right? You're not a husband or a father, nor do you want to be. But that's what I can't understand. Because the Kiernan I know is kind and compassionate. He's someone who goes the extra mile for his patients, but he also cares about the people in his life. Think about how you cancelled a surgery to stay with me when you knew I was upset. Or how you wouldn't let me leave the hospital and comforted me when I had an anxiety attack after visiting the birthing suite."

Claire's words had nearly knocked Kiernan backwards, but she wasn't finished.

"You're not your father, Kiernan. Yet for some inexplicable reason, you seem convinced that you are. And you know what the saddest part of all this is?"

Kiernan wasn't sure, but he was pretty damn certain that Claire was about to tell him.

"The person you're hurting the most is yourself. Because I *know* you would be an amazing father and husband. And if you could only get past whatever it is that has you convinced otherwise, I know you'd find happiness in committing to more than just your career. And I mean a different kind of happiness—not the one you can find in your work, no matter how dedicated you are or how many lives you save."

It was only the sensation of raindrops on his bottom lip that made Kiernan realize his mouth was slightly agape. He swallowed to close it.

"I think I'm having one of those sorry-not-sorry moments," Claire said sheepishly, as though she, too, was shocked by her own words. "I wasn't actually planning to say all of that. It just kind of came out."

It took several moments for Kiernan to reply, "That's okay." He knew how insufficient those two words were at a moment like this, but was too paralyzed to say anything more.

As Claire reached over and clasped his hand he

shuddered at her touch—and at the thought that he might never feel the warmth of her skin again.

"What I *did* come here to say is that I think it's best if we say goodbye now…before it gets even harder to do so. At least harder for me."

"Claire…"

She stared at him, clearly waiting for him to say more. But as the world around him seemingly came to a halt, he could only pose two questions in his mind. Could this be it? Was it the last time he would ever look into her eyes? He'd known this day was coming—but not here…not in this very moment.

Say something!

His directive fell on deaf ears—*his* deaf ears. No, that wasn't quite right. He heard himself, loud and clear, but what could he say? That she was right and he *was* missing out on the joy of having a partner in life and children? *Was* she right?

His breath choked in his throat. It was all too much to take in at this moment. Still, there was something he needed to know.

"Will you be going back to Boston General?"

Claire briefly looked down at the ground, but not before he saw disappointment in her eyes. Was she hoping that he'd tell her she was right, rather than ask about her career decision? He had only asked because he desperately wanted her to continue the work she was meant to do.

Claire looked back up at him. "I might not return to the hospital itself, given that I think a fresh start somewhere else will probably be better for me. But I also think I've come to realize over the last few weeks that making a difference in the lives of mothers and their babies is the work that I'm meant to do." She stared earnestly into Kiernan's eyes. "And I have you to thank for that."

"Claire—"

She squeezed his hand. "I'm not sure what the medical equivalent is of getting back in the saddle…"

A half-smile emerged on Kiernan's lips. "Getting back into the scrubs?"

She grinned. "Something like that. But without your encouragement and support I never would have been able to do it."

"You're an incredible doctor—all I did was open the door. You're the one who willingly walked through it, despite what I know had to be immense difficulty in doing so. I'm just so grateful and proud of you that you did."

With a surge of wind, the drizzle turned into steady rain that began to drum down upon them. Kiernan looked up at the sky, only to be immediately pelted in the eyes.

Claire looked up as well. "Where's an umbrella when you need one?"

Kiernan studied her closely through the raindrops that were pooling on his eyelashes. Even with her hair plastered against the sides of her face and rivulets of water running down her nose and cheeks, she was exquisitely beautiful, both inside and out.

"Come on," he said. "Let's go inside."

"Actually, I think I'll go back to my cottage."

Right, Kiernan thought, his stomach sinking. And it wasn't alone. His heart also plunged as reality set in. *This is the end of the road for us. And it's my doing.*

"Let me at least drive you back."

He hoped beyond hope that she'd take up his offer—if for no other reason than to avoid the rain. At least he would have another ten minutes in her presence.

"No—I'm fine. It's not a long walk. And, believe it or not, I sometimes like being out in the rain."

There it was again. The streak of stubbornness and independence that drove him crazy, but also garnered his admiration.

"Take care of yourself, Kiernan," Claire said, her voice subdued and yet almost echoing against the roar of the rain. "I'll never forget the time that we spent together."

One more long, lingering look his way, and then she turned and walked away from him along the pier. He was still watching intently as she turned left onto the perpendicular portion of the platform that led back to the shore, knowing she would then take the paved path beside the road that led to her cottage.

Soon she disappeared from view. And still, he stayed.

Another ten minutes passed—or was it more like fifteen? Kiernan couldn't be sure. He continued to stare off into the distance, only vaguely aware of the slightly swaying pier beneath his feet as the storm-provoked winds and waves kicked into overdrive.

Apparently he must like the rain, too, he thought. Because here he was, soaked to the bone and then some, and still he couldn't step away from the last spot where he had held Claire's hands and stared into her eyes.

Back at his home, later that night, Kiernan leaned up against the deck railing and stared outwards. He usually did his best thinking when it was just him and the endless expanse of ocean, but now its powers of insight seemed to be on hold. Never in a million years had he thought he'd be facing such a seemingly insurmountable impasse...

But *was* it insurmountable?

Since his early teens, he'd had his whole life mapped out before him. Perhaps it had been a way to assert control when everything else around him at the time had seemed to be about as stable and solid as quicksand. And there was no doubt that this steely resolve had served him well over the years. It had got him through medical school when his own father had cast doubts on his ability to succeed. And it had kept him rising up the ranks as a surgeon, culminating in a position that would allow him to have the greatest impact on patients in need of potentially life-saving care.

But at what cost?

Kiernan shook his head, dumbfounded by his own question. He had never dared ask himself this before—simply because it was a non-issue.

Meeting Claire had changed all of that.

Like a kaleidoscope of images, every moment spent with Claire played out in his mind. From performing a high-risk delivery together, as two strangers in the back of an ambulance, to their passionate encounter in the castle and everything in between… In less than a month she had managed to capture his heart in a way that no other woman ever had. And now he was losing her. Not only to her inevitable return to America, but to his rigid insistence that children were not part of his life plan.

You can break the cycle, you know.

Claire's earlier words echoed in his mind. Was it possible that he had been denying himself the joy and fulfillment of having a family of his own all because of his negative experiences as the son of a negligent father? It couldn't be that simple—a textbook case of unintentionally sabotaging his own ultimate happiness due to the misdeeds of his dad.

It just couldn't.

Or…could it?

"I am not my father," he said quietly into the wind.

It whistled back, as though reassuring him that his thoughts were the key to his salvation.

Nothing would make him happier than seeing Claire with the child that she so desperately wanted. A child that would help heal the wounds of her past loss. A child that she would love with the endless compassion that was so much a part of who she was.

There was only one problem. He couldn't imagine her sharing that joy with anyone but him.

The revelation frightened him—but not because it meant upending a life plan that up until very recently had been set in immovable stone. No, the fear was that it was too late to reverse course. Claire was leaving the country on Saturday. That gave him three days to do…*something*. And it had to be big.

His mind whirled and whirled and whirled.

Yes…yes…uh-huh…right.

Another nod as a plan emerged out of thin air and began to take shape in his thoughts.

It was crazy. *He* was crazy.

The formerly logical, even-keeled, uber-grounded surgeon was about to go off the deep end, and he had zero regrets. His only regret would be if he waited another second and ended up being too late.

It was time to set his plan in motion.

CHAPTER THIRTEEN

CLAIRE TOSSED SOME cracked corn to the ducks as she walked along the shoreline behind her cottage. Earlier in the day she had started to pack for her inevitable flight home tomorrow, but hadn't got any further than throwing a pair of jeans and two tops into the suitcase.

She didn't have to look deep within herself to know that her heart wasn't fully on board with returning to Boston. Nor did she have to question why. Or, more precisely, the *who* behind the why.

Still, she didn't regret a single second that she had spent with Kiernan. *Not one.* In so many ways he had helped her heal from a loss that had previously seemed insurmountable. She would never, ever forget precious Ariana, but the thoughts were no longer paralyzing to her very soul like they had been before. Plus, she was ready to reengage in her career as an ob-gyn—another step forward that only a month ago had seemed impossible.

And he showed you that you can fall in love again.

Claire winced. If ever there was a positive that came with an equally weighted negative, this had to be it. Yes, she now knew she could love again.

But she could love *Kiernan*—a distinction that was non-negotiable. And now, she had to leave him.

Even if you stayed, you'd still have to say good-bye.

Claire pressed her lips together, jaw tightened. Did she really need to remind herself of the obvious?

Just be glad for the time you had together, she told herself.

Not *too* much of cliché, she thought, but it was a notion she was going to hold on to…because right now it was all she had.

"I thought I might find you here."

Claire gasped and whirled around, her eyes wide with disbelief as she saw Kiernan standing barely ten feet away from her. He wore a grin that suited his handsome face in the same way that his dark jeans and long-sleeved burgundy T-shirt suited his muscular body.

It took a few moments for Claire to process what was happening. She had told Kiernan no more goodbyes. But, damn, was she ever happy that he had ignored her request.

"I had to see you again," he said as he walked over and took both her hands in his. "So please don't get mad at me for defying your orders."

She couldn't help but laugh quietly at his cheekiness. "That's okay. I'm supposed to be packing to leave, but as you can see, I've been procrastinating." As he squeezed her hands and pulled her in closer, she could feel the electricity surge between them. "And I can think of worse diversions than seeing you again."

He smiled, but then his face grew serious. "Claire, I couldn't let you leave without telling you something."

She waited for him to continue, suddenly aware that she was holding her breath.

"I love you," he said softly. "And in a way that I've never loved anyone before. You are the most gifted, caring, beautiful...*amazing* woman, and you've made me see things that no one else ever has. Or ever could. Being with you has made me a better person. Which I know probably sounds crazy, given that we've only known each other a month. But it's been a month that's completely changed my life."

Claire caught her breath just in time before it escaped her once more. "I love you, too," she said quietly. "Which is why saying goodbye is so hard..."

"But what if we didn't have to say goodbye?"

Her forehead creased in confusion. They had been over this before. Surely he knew why they had to part ways.

Realizing there was no point in repeating their conflicting views on family, she could only look at him with questioning eyes.

"I've been doing a lot of thinking over the past few days," he said. "*A lot.* You said something to me that day we went hiking. How I could be the one to break the cycle. At the time I knew what you meant on an intellectual level, but I couldn't truly *feel* it, if you know what I mean. But I do now. My desire not to have kids totally stemmed from my father's inadequacies. I thought that being the best surgeon I could be meant forgoing a family, or else being an absentee husband and father like him. But it's simply not true. Being with you…it's made me see what really matters in life. The work that we both do as doctors—yes, that is important. It can even save lives. But it's not the be-all and end-all. I want to spend the rest of my life with you. And to have a family together."

He looked up at the sky, shaking his head and nearly laughing, as though he couldn't comprehend how some of his core beliefs had suddenly been turned upside down.

"All of my life I've wanted to steer clear of anything that remotely hinted at having a family of my own. And now…because of you…it's like I suddenly can't think about anything else."

"Kiernan… I…"

Was this really happening?

She swallowed hard, reminding herself that she needed to stay grounded in reality. "You do know that I'm flying back to Boston tomorrow."

"I know. But I also know that you probably won't be going back to Boston General—at least that's what you shared with me. So I hope you don't mind that I took the liberty of making a few inquiries."

Claire arched an eyebrow. "A few inquiries…?"

"I've been in talks with the hospital board and the CEO, and they all agree. There's no one more qualified to lead West Mercy's new neonatal wing than you. They're still hammering out the fine print, but if you're interested they're prepared to offer you a contract that will give you full control over the direction of this new program. Fetal surgeries, treatments for high-risk mothers—all of it."

Claire didn't think her jaw could fall any further, but with this most unexpected announcement, it found a way. Her mind, though spinning, travelled back to a recent wish…a seemingly *impossible* wish…that she was living in the beautiful Irish countryside and working with the love of her life, who just so happened to be gazing into her eyes at this very moment.

And now Kiernan was pledging his love to her and sharing his desire for them to have a family together. Which meant that in the span of a single minute—two at tops—he had just made all her dreams come true.

"I know this is a lot to throw at you all at once," he said. "And I don't want you to feel in any way pressured to make a decision now. Take whatever time you need. Go home, like you planned, and talk to your family about it if that helps." He paused. "Oh—and I should mention that the contract comes with a very important rider."

Seeing the glint of a twinkle in his eye, Claire grinned cautiously as she asked, "Which is…?"

"Twenty-four-seven access to the chief of surgery, who is fully invested in the goal of making you the happiest woman on earth."

"You've already done that," Claire said softly as Kiernan leaned in and kissed her passionately.

"Like I said before," Kiernan said, once they both had a chance to breathe again. "No pressure... But while you're tossing around the pros and cons of my offer, how about we go inside the cottage and I'll show you some of the exclusive benefits you'll get with that contract rider?"

Claire grinned. She already knew what her answer would be, but there was no need to let the chief of surgery know just yet. "Okay... But just so you know—I'm very much on the fence about this offer, so you'll really need to persuade me."

His eyes flashed with desire as they gazed into hers. "Oh, I will... I can promise you that."

Claire had no doubt Kiernan would keep his promise. He was just that kind of man.

EPILOGUE

CLAIRE PROPPED HERSELF up on both elbows as she lay down on a soft blanket covering an equally cushiony carpet of grass. The early-afternoon sun felt good on her face, and with her eyes closed, she tipped her head back.

"Nothing like getting some vitamin D the good, old-fashioned way."

Kiernan leaned over and kissed her on the forehead. "Hard to believe that exactly one year ago we met at this precise spot."

Claire opened her eyes and smiled. "I know. I sometimes wonder…what if I'd come here for a walk twenty minutes sooner, or you'd gone for a run twenty minutes later. Chances are we never would have met."

"Or been at the right place, at the right time, to help deliver Sam."

"Exactly."

"So, are you saying you believe in fate?" Kiernan asked, with a teasing quality to his voice.

Claire smiled wistfully. "Either that or extremely good luck."

Kiernan scanned the grass that lined the border of the blanket, then plucked a four-leaf clover. He offered it to Claire, placing his other hand on her belly. "Well, I can personally vouch for the fact that I'm the luckiest man alive."

She placed her hand over his. At four and a half months pregnant, she had just started to experience Caitlin's kicks, and her smile widened as one poked her just under her ribcage.

"Did you feel that?" she asked excitedly.

Kiernan nodded, his face beaming with pride. "I think we have a star football player in the making. Or, better yet, a rugby player."

A ringing phone interrupted Claire's laughter.

"Who is it?" she asked as Kiernan glanced down at his phone screen.

"It's Craig," he replied, rolling his eyes.

Two more rings, and the call stopped.

"You can call him back. I don't mind."

"It's nothing that can't wait."

"Are you sure about that? You don't want the hospital CEO labeling you a slacker." She paused. "And I'm only half kidding, by the way, knowing how he expects twenty-four-seven access."

"It's a beautiful Saturday afternoon, and I'm here with my even more beautiful wife. If it were a medical emergency, I'd take the call. But administrative stuff—that can wait until Monday."

"You really have become quite the slouch, Mr. O'Rourke."

Kiernan grinned. "If it means spending more time with you and our daughter, then I'll gladly own up to that."

"I love you," she said, at the exact moment Kiernan uttered the same three words.

They both laughed at the unintended perfect timing.

"And I can't wait to meet you, little Caitlin," Kiernan said as he leaned over and kissed her belly.

Claire lifted the four-leaf clover that she had been twirling between her thumb and forefinger and studied it for a moment. There had to be some truth to its powers of good fortune. Because she was, indeed, the luckiest woman in the world.

* * * * *